# The ULTIMATE
# CHAIR YOGA
## Guide for Seniors
## Over 60

---

Practical and Simple 28-day Chair Yoga Plan
for Seniors - Build Strength, Increase Flexibility
and Manage Weight

ARDEN COOPER

Legal Notice

The information provided in this book is for general informational purposes only and is not intended as legal, medical, or professional advice. The author and publisher of this book make no representations or warranties with respect to the accuracy, applicability, or completeness of the contents of this book. They disclaim any responsibility for any liability, loss, or risk, personal or otherwise, which is incurred as a consequence, directly or indirectly, of the use and application of any of the contents of this book.

Disclaimer

The material in this book is provided for informational purposes only and is not intended to be a substitute for professional medical advice, diagnosis, or treatment. Always seek the advice of your physician or other qualified health provider with any questions you may have regarding a medical condition. Never disregard professional medical advice or delay in seeking it because of something you have read in this book. Reliance on any information provided in this book is solely at your own risk.

# CONTENTS

## CHAPTER 07. The Ultimate 28-Day Chair Yoga Plan  67

# CHAPTER 08. Staying Motivated    79

## CHAPTER 09. Chair Yoga Beyond the Basics    87

# INTRODUCTION

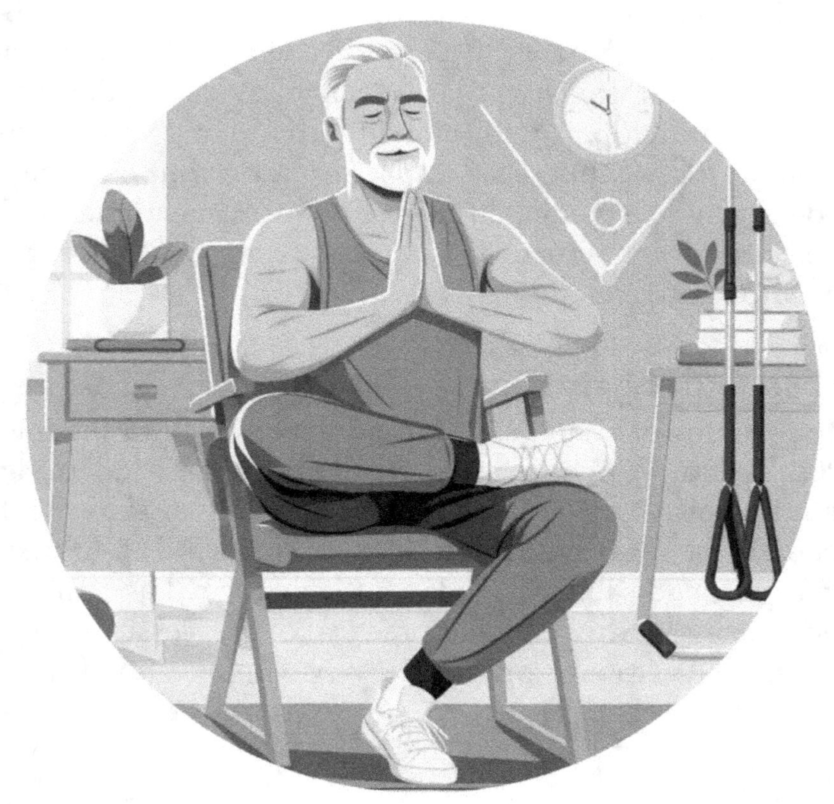

Welcome to **"The Ultimate Chair Yoga Guide for Seniors Over 60"!** In this comprehensive guide, we'll explore the wonderful world of chair yoga and its numerous benefits for seniors. Whether you're new to yoga or a seasoned practitioner looking for a gentle practice, chair yoga offers a safe, accessible, and effective way to improve your health and well-being.

# Introduction to Chair Yoga

Chair yoga is a modified form of yoga that adapts traditional yoga poses to be performed while seated or using a chair for support. It's an excellent option for seniors, individuals with mobility limitations, or anyone looking for a gentle, low-impact exercise routine. Chair yoga combines gentle stretches, mindful breathing, and relaxation techniques to promote flexibility, strength, balance, and overall vitality.

## History of Chair Yoga

The origins of chair yoga can be traced back to the late 20th century when yoga teachers began adapting traditional yoga poses for individuals who couldn't participate in a regular mat-based practice due to age, injury, or disability. Today, chair yoga has gained popularity worldwide as a practical and accessible form of yoga that can be practiced by people of all ages and abilities.

# Benefits of Chair Yoga for Seniors

Chair yoga offers a wide range of benefits for seniors, both physically and mentally. Here are some of the key benefits you can expect to experience:

### 1. Improved Balance and Flexibility

Chair yoga helps improve balance and flexibility by gently stretching and lengthening muscles, tendons, and ligaments. By practicing a variety of seated and standing poses, you'll increase your range of motion and reduce the risk of falls and injuries.

## 2. Increased Strength and Range of Motion

Chair yoga poses are designed to strengthen muscles throughout the body, including the core, arms, legs, and back. Regular practice helps build muscular strength and endurance, enhancing overall stability and mobility.

## 3. Reduced Pain and Stiffness

Chair yoga can help alleviate chronic pain and stiffness associated with conditions such as arthritis, back pain, and fibromyalgia. Gentle stretches and movements improve circulation, reduce inflammation, and promote relaxation, leading to decreased pain and discomfort.

## 4. Improved Mood and Well-being

Chair yoga incorporates mindfulness and relaxation techniques that promote mental and emotional well-being. By focusing on the present moment and connecting with your breath, you'll experience reduced stress, anxiety, and depression, and an increased sense of peace and contentment.

## 5. Boosted Heart Health

Chair yoga promotes cardiovascular health by improving circulation, lowering blood pressure, and reducing the risk of heart disease. Gentle movements and deep breathing exercises help strengthen the heart muscle and improve overall cardiovascular function.

# Setting Realistic Expectations and Goals

As you embark on your chair yoga journey, it's essential to set realistic expectations and goals for yourself. Remember that yoga is a personal practice, and progress looks different for everyone. Here are some tips for setting realistic expectations and goals:

## 1. Start Slow

If you're new to yoga or have physical limitations, start with gentle, beginner-friendly poses and gradually increase the intensity and duration of your practice as you feel more comfortable.

## 2. Listen to Your Body

Pay attention to how your body feels during and after each practice session. Honor your limitations and avoid pushing yourself beyond what feels safe and comfortable. Modify poses as needed to suit your individual needs and abilities.

## 3. Be Patient and Persistent

Rome wasn't built in a day, and neither is your yoga practice. Progress takes time, so be patient with yourself and trust the process. Stay consistent with your practice, even on days when you don't feel like it, and you'll gradually see improvements over time.

## 4. Focus on Non-Physical Benefits

While physical improvements are often the most visible, don't overlook the non-physical benefits of chair yoga, such as reduced stress, improved mood, and enhanced overall well-being. These benefits are just as valuable, if not more so, than the physical ones.

By setting realistic expectations and goals for your chair yoga practice, you'll create a positive and sustainable foundation for long-term growth and transformation. Remember that the journey is just as important as the destination, so enjoy the process, stay open to new experiences, and embrace the power of chair yoga to enrich your life.

In the chapters that follow, we'll dive deeper into the various aspects of chair yoga, including basic poses, breathing techniques, safety tips, and more. Whether you're looking to improve your balance, increase your flexibility, or simply enjoy a moment of relaxation, there's something for everyone in "The Ultimate Chair Yoga Guide for Seniors Over 60". Let's begin our journey together towards health, happiness, and vitality!

# Chapter 01

## Getting Started with Chair Yoga

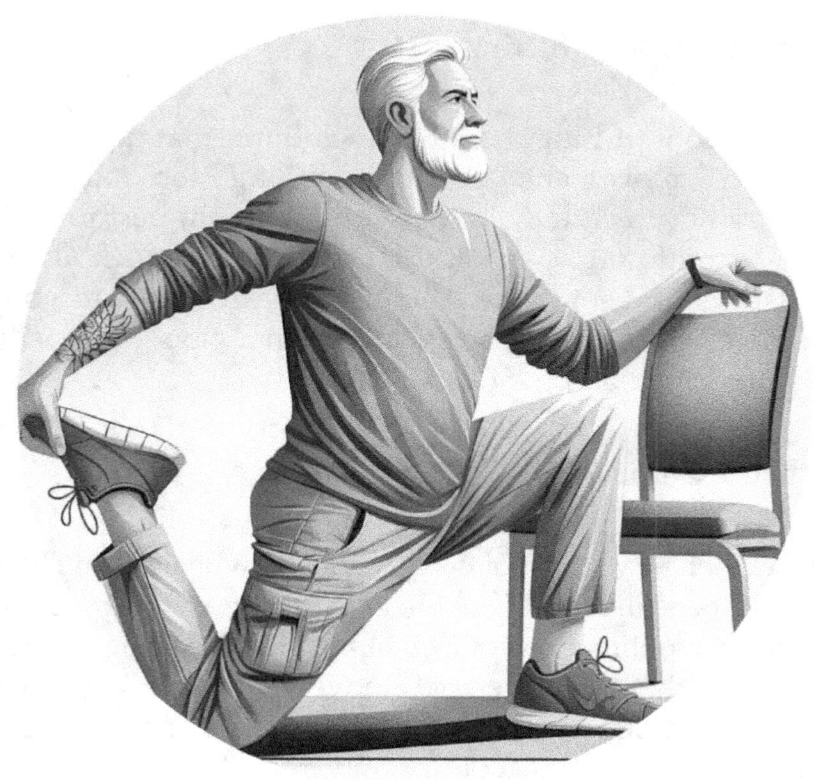

In this chapter, we'll lay the foundation for your chair yoga journey, covering everything from what you'll need to get started to important safety tips and basic breathing techniques.

# What You'll Need to Get Started

Before diving into chair yoga, it's essential to gather a few items to ensure a comfortable and safe practice:

## Comfortable Clothing

Choose loose-fitting, breathable clothing that allows for ease of movement. Avoid anything too tight or constricting, as it may hinder your ability to perform the poses comfortably. Look for fabrics that wick away moisture to keep you feeling fresh throughout your practice. Consider wearing layers that you can easily remove if you become too warm.

## Sturdy Chair

Select a chair with a solid back and no wheels. The chair should be stable and capable of supporting your weight without wobbling. Avoid chairs with arms that are too high, as they may restrict movement during certain poses. Additionally, ensure that the chair is at a height where your feet can comfortably rest flat on the floor with your knees bent at a 90-degree angle.

# What to Wear for Chair Yoga

The key to dressing for chair yoga is comfort and flexibility. Here are some tips on what to wear:

- **Stretchy Fabrics:** Opt for materials that stretch and move with your body, such as cotton or spandex blends. These fabrics allow for unrestricted movement and won't constrict you during poses.
- **Layers:** Dress in layers that you can easily remove if you become too warm during your practice. This allows you to adjust your clothing based on your comfort level and the temperature of your practice space.
- **Comfortable Shoes:** While chair yoga is typically done barefoot or in socks, you may want to wear supportive shoes if you have foot pain or balance issues. Choose shoes with a non-slip sole to ensure stability during standing poses.

# Setting Up Your Practice Space

Creating a conducive environment for your chair yoga practice is essential for maximizing relaxation and focus. Follow these guidelines when setting up your practice space:

## Quiet Environment

Choose a quiet area free from distractions where you can focus solely on your practice. This might mean finding a secluded corner of your home or setting aside a dedicated yoga space where you can practice without interruptions. Consider playing soft instrumental music or nature sounds to enhance relaxation and drown out background noise.

## Well-Lit Area

Ensure adequate lighting in the room to prevent eye strain and enhance visibility during poses. Natural light is ideal, but if that's not available, use soft, diffused lighting that illuminates the space evenly. Position your chair near a window or under a bright overhead light to make it easier to see your movements and maintain proper alignment.

## Comfortable Seating

Place your chair on a non-slip surface and adjust its position to maintain good posture throughout your practice. The chair should be stable and level, with all four legs making contact with the floor. If necessary, place a yoga mat or non-skid rug pad beneath the chair to prevent it from sliding during dynamic movements.

# Important Safety Tips

Safety is paramount in any exercise routine, especially for seniors. Here are some crucial safety tips to keep in mind during your chair yoga practice:

## Listen to Your Body

Pay attention to how your body feels during each pose. If you experience pain or discomfort, ease out of the pose and modify it as needed. Pushing through pain can lead to injury and may exacerbate existing conditions. Remember that yoga is about honoring your body's limitations and finding a balance between effort and ease.

## When to Modify or Avoid Poses

Not all poses may be suitable for everyone, especially seniors or individuals with pre-existing health conditions. Listen to your body and modify or skip poses that feel too challenging or cause discomfort. Common modifications include using props like blocks or blankets to support your body, reducing the range of motion in a pose, or choosing alternative poses that target the same muscle groups.

## Stay Hydrated

Maintaining proper hydration is essential, even during a low-impact activity like chair yoga. Keep a water bottle nearby and sip water throughout your practice to prevent dehydration. Aim to drink at least 8 ounces of water before starting your practice and continue hydrating as needed during breaks or whenever you feel thirsty. Dehydration can lead to fatigue, dizziness, and muscle cramps, so it's crucial to stay hydrated to support your overall well-being.

## Warm Up and Cool Down

Before starting your chair yoga practice, take a few minutes to warm up your body with gentle movements and stretches. This helps increase blood flow to your muscles, lubricate your joints, and prepare your body for more intense activity. Similarly, at the end of your practice, take time to cool down with calming stretches and deep breathing exercises to relax your muscles and promote recovery. Skipping warm-up and cool-down activities increases your risk of injury and may leave you feeling stiff or sore afterward.

# Basic Breathing Techniques

Breath is a fundamental aspect of yoga practice, helping to calm the mind and enhance relaxation. One of the foundational breathing techniques in chair yoga is deep diaphragmatic breathing:

1. **Find a Comfortable Seated Position:** Sit upright in your chair with your feet flat on the floor and hands resting on your thighs. Close your eyes if it feels comfortable or soften your gaze downward to reduce visual distractions.
2. **Relax Your Shoulders:** Roll your shoulders back and down, allowing them to rest comfortably away from your ears. Feel the lengthening of your spine as you sit tall and proud, maintaining a sense of openness in your chest and shoulders.
3. **Inhale Slowly Through Your Nose:** Take a slow, deep breath in through your nose, allowing your abdomen to expand as you fill your lungs with air. Feel the breath moving down into your belly, ribcage, and upper chest, creating a sense of expansion and spaciousness within your body.
4. **Exhale Slowly Through Your Mouth:** Release the breath slowly through your mouth, contracting your abdomen gently to expel all the air. Notice the

sensation of your belly drawing inward as you release the breath, feeling a sense of grounding and relaxation with each exhale.

5. **Repeat Several Times:** Continue this deep breathing pattern for several rounds, focusing on the sensation of the breath filling your body with each inhale and releasing tension with each exhale. Allow your breath to become slow, steady, and rhythmic, syncing up with the natural pace of your body's movements.

Practice this basic breathing technique regularly to cultivate a sense of calm and relaxation in your chair yoga practice. As you become more familiar with deep diaphragmatic breathing, you can explore other breathwork techniques to deepen your practice and enhance your overall well-being.

With these foundational elements in place, you're ready to embark on your chair yoga journey with confidence and ease. In the following chapters, we'll delve deeper into specific poses and sequences to help you build strength, increase flexibility, and manage weight effectively. Whether you're a beginner or an experienced practitioner, chair yoga offers a gentle yet powerful way to improve your physical health, mental well-being, and overall quality of life. Get ready to experience the transformative benefits of this accessible and enjoyable practice as we explore the diverse world of chair yoga together.

# Chapter 02

## Basic Chair Yoga Poses

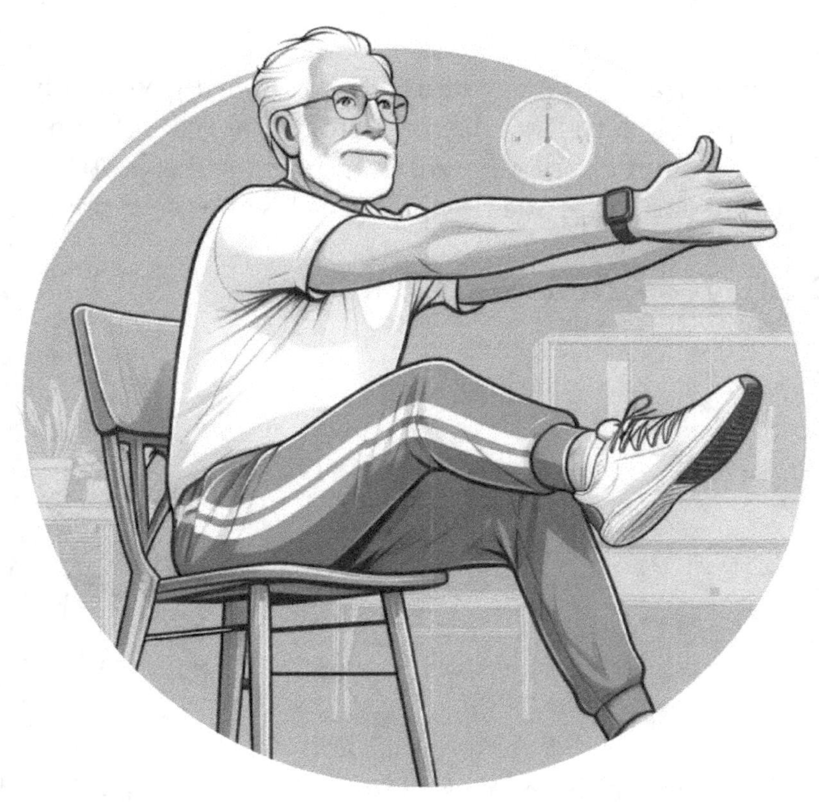

In this chapter, we'll explore a series of basic chair yoga poses designed to gently stretch and strengthen your body. These poses are suitable for beginners and can be modified to accommodate various levels of flexibility and mobility. We'll begin with a warm-up sequence to prepare your body for movement and conclude with a relaxing cool-down to help you unwind and release tension.

# Warm-up

A proper warm-up is essential for preparing your body for physical activity and reducing the risk of injury. These gentle movements will help increase blood flow to your muscles, improve flexibility, and enhance mobility.

## Gentle Neck Rolls

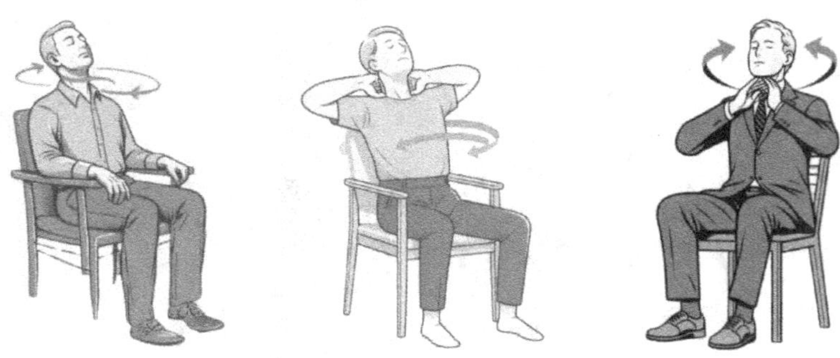

1. Sit comfortably in your chair with your spine tall and your shoulders relaxed.
2. Inhale as you gently tilt your head to the right, bringing your right ear towards your right shoulder.
3. Exhale as you roll your chin towards your chest,

feeling a gentle stretch along the left side of your neck.

4. Inhale as you continue rolling your head to the left, bringing your left ear towards your left shoulder.
5. Exhale as you roll your chin back towards your chest, completing a full circle with your neck.
6. Repeat this movement in the opposite direction, rolling your head from left to right.
7. Continue alternating between clockwise and counterclockwise neck rolls for several repetitions, moving slowly and mindfully.

## Shoulder Rolls

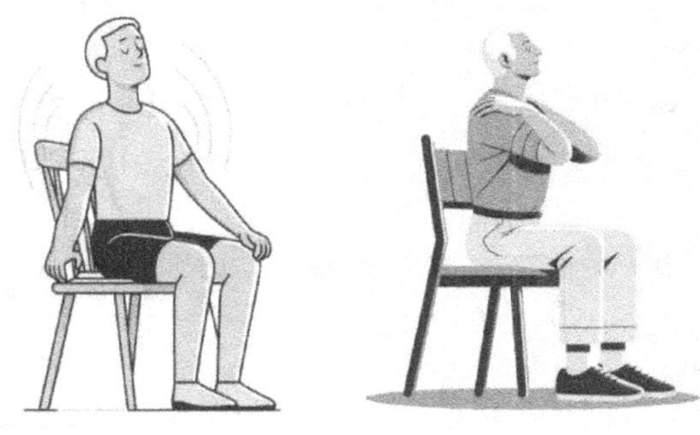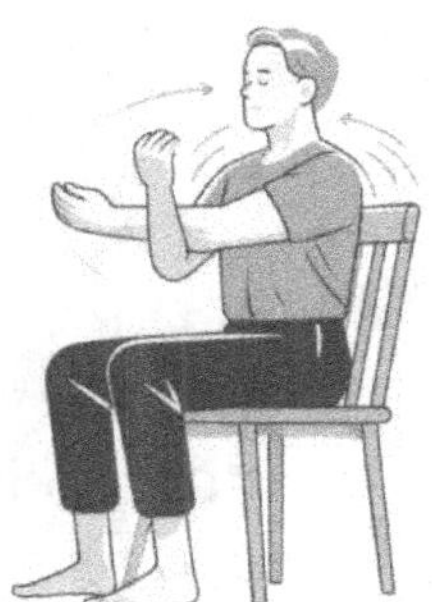

1. Sit tall in your chair with your fe5et flat on the floor and your hands resting on your thighs.
2. Inhale as you lift your shoulders up towards your ears, feeling a gentle stretch across your upper back.
3. Exhale as you roll your shoulders back and down in a smooth, circular motion, squeezing your shoulder blades together.
4. Continue rolling your shoulders in this circular motion for several repetitions, focusing on releasing

tension and opening up your chest.

## Arm Circles (Forward and Backward)

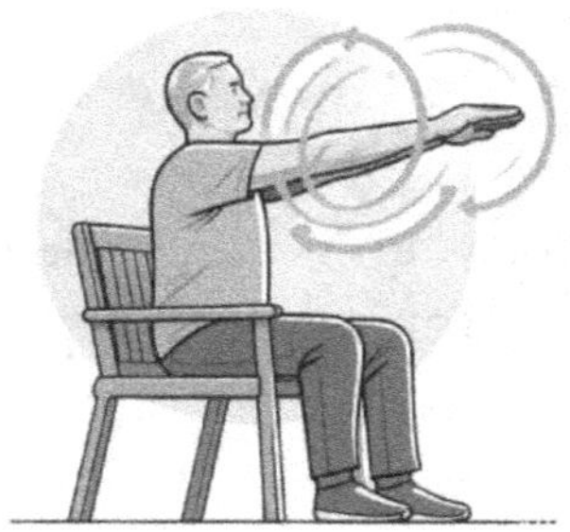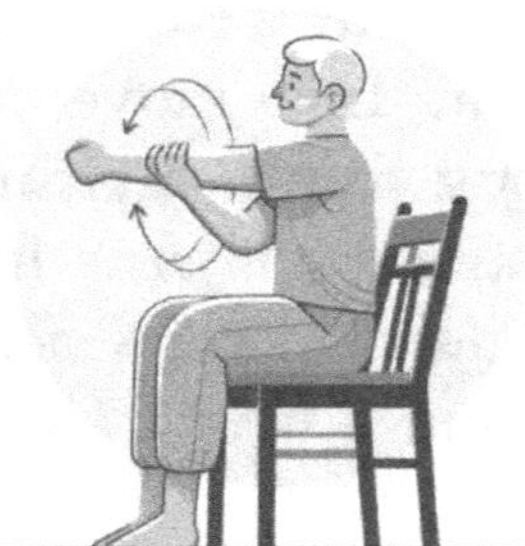

1. Extend your arms out to the sides at shoulder height, palms facing down.
2. Inhale as you sweep your arms forward and up towards the ceiling, bringing your palms together overhead.
3. Exhale as you lower your arms back down to shoulder height, opening your chest and spreading your fingers wide.
4. Repeat this movement for several repetitions, flowing smoothly between arm circles.
5. After completing forward arm circles, reverse the motion and perform backward arm circles, sweeping your arms back and down behind you.
6. Focus on maintaining a steady breath and fluid movement throughout the exercise, keeping your shoulders relaxed and your spine tall.

## Seated Torso Twists

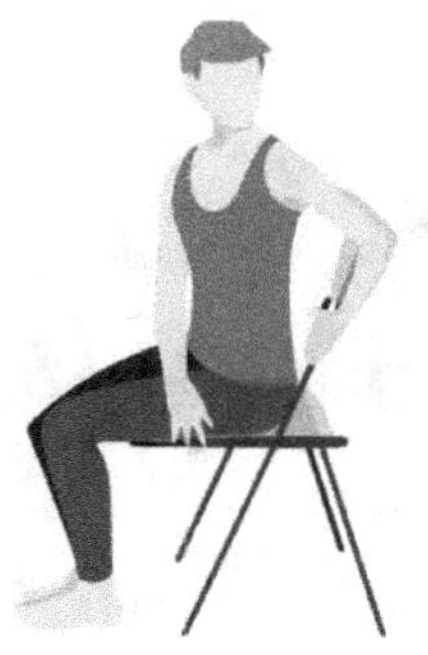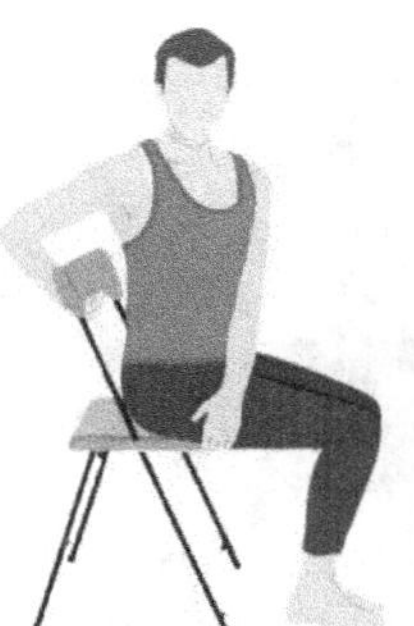

1.  Sit tall in your chair with your feet flat on the floor and your hands resting on your thighs.
2.  Inhale as you lengthen your spine, lifting through the crown of your head.
3.  Exhale as you twist your torso to the right, placing your left hand on the outside of your right thigh and your right hand on the back of the chair.
4.  Inhale to lengthen your spine and deepen the twist, turning your gaze over your right shoulder.
5.  Exhale as you release the twist and return to center.
6.  Repeat the twist to the left side, placing your right hand on the outside of your left thigh and your left hand on the back of the chair.
7.  Inhale to lengthen your spine and deepen the twist, turning your gaze over your left shoulder.
8.  Exhale as you release the twist and return to center.
9.  Continue alternating between right and left torso twists for several repetitions, moving with your breath and maintaining a smooth, controlled movement.

## Ankle Circles

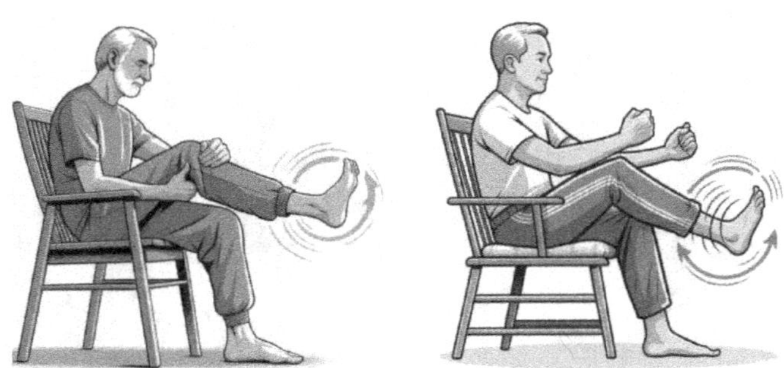

1. Sit comfortably in your chair with your feet flat on the floor.
2. Lift your right foot off the floor and begin tracing circles with your toes, moving in a clockwise direction.
3. Focus on making slow, controlled movements, articulating through your ankle joint to create full circles.
4. After several repetitions, reverse the direction of the circles and trace them in a counterclockwise motion.
5. Repeat the ankle circles with your left foot, first in a clockwise direction and then in a counterclockwise direction.
6. Continue alternating between right and left ankle circles for several repetitions, moving mindfully and maintaining steady breathing throughout.

# Cool-down

After completing the warm-up sequence, it's important to take time to cool down and relax your body. These seated stretches and relaxation techniques will help you release tension and promote a sense of calm and well-being.

## Seated Forward Bends

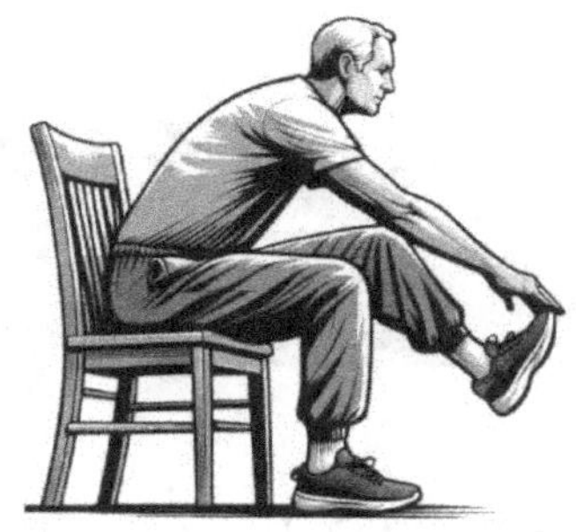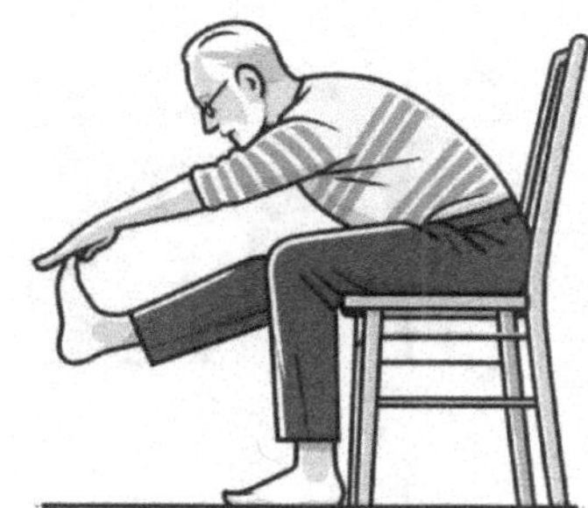

1. Sit tall in your chair with your feet flat on the floor and your hands resting on your thighs.
2. Inhale as you lengthen your spine, lifting through the crown of your head.
3. Exhale as you hinge forward at your hips, leading with your chest and reaching your hands towards your feet.
4. Keep your spine long and your shoulders relaxed as you fold forward, feeling a gentle stretch along the back of your legs and spine.
5. Hold the forward bend for several breaths, breathing deeply into any areas of tension or tightness.
6. On an inhale, slowly rise back up to a seated position,

stacking your vertebrae one at a time.

7. Repeat the seated forward bend for several repetitions, moving with your breath and gradually increasing the depth of the stretch with each repetition.

## Seated Side Stretches

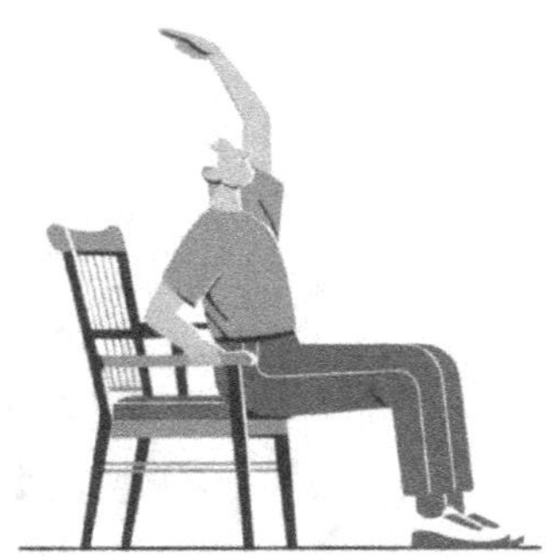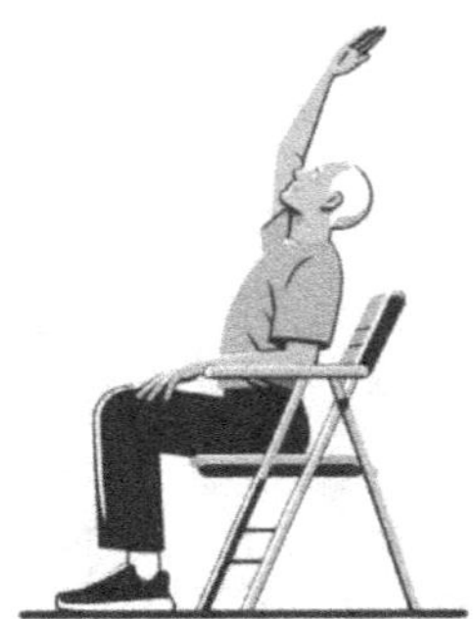

1. Sit tall in your chair with your feet flat on the floor and your hands resting on your thighs.
2. Inhale as you lengthen your spine, lifting through the crown of your head.
3. Exhale as you reach your right arm overhead, stretching up and over to the left side of your body.
4. Keep both hips grounded on the chair as you lengthen through your right side, feeling a gentle stretch from your fingertips to your hip.
5. Hold the side stretch for several breaths, breathing deeply into the space between your ribs.
6. On an inhale, slowly release the stretch and return to center.
7. Repeat the side stretch on the opposite side, reaching your left arm overhead and stretching up and over to

the right side of your body.

8.  Hold the stretch for several breaths, focusing on creating length and space along your left side.
9.  Continue alternating between right and left side stretches for several repetitions, moving with your breath and maintaining a steady, rhythmic pace.

# Deep Breaths and Relaxation Techniques

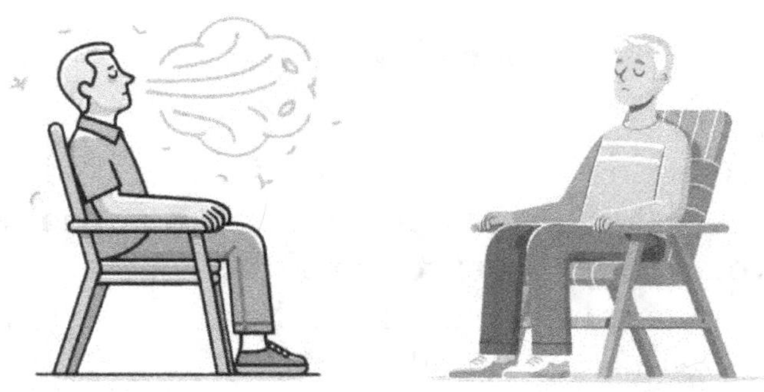

1.  Sit comfortably in your chair with your feet flat on the floor and your hands resting on your thighs.
2.  Close your eyes or soften your gaze downward to reduce visual distractions.
3.  Take a few moments to focus on your breath, noticing the natural rhythm of inhalation and exhalation.
4.  Inhale deeply through your nose, feeling your belly expand with each breath.
5.  Exhale slowly through your mouth, releasing any tension or stress with each breath.
6.  Continue this deep breathing pattern for several minutes, allowing your breath to become slow,

steady, and effortless.

7. As you breathe, imagine each inhale filling you with energy and vitality, while each exhale releases any negativity or fatigue.

8. Allow yourself to sink into a state of deep relaxation, surrendering to the present moment and letting go of any worries or distractions.

9. When you're ready, gently open your eyes and take a moment to notice how you feel, appreciating the sense of calm and tranquility that fills your body and mind.

# Conclusion

Congratulations! You've completed a series of basic chair yoga poses designed to gently stretch, strengthen, and relax your body. Incorporating these poses into your daily routine can help improve flexibility, mobility, and overall well-being. Whether you're new to yoga or a seasoned practitioner, chair yoga offers a safe and accessible way to enhance your physical and mental health. In the following chapters, we'll explore more advanced poses and sequences to further deepen your practice and support your journey towards optimal health and vitality. Get ready to experience the transformative benefits of chair yoga as we continue to explore this enriching practice together.

# Chapter 03

## Building a Strong Foundation - Core and Leg Exercises

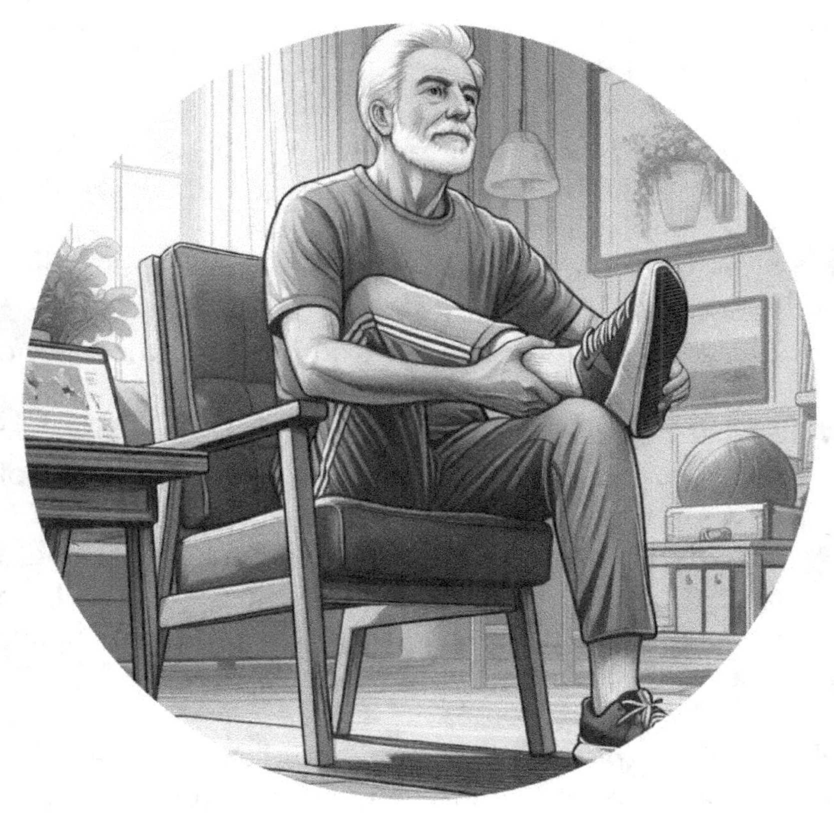

In this chapter, we'll focus on building a strong foundation through core and leg exercises specifically tailored for seniors. These exercises target key muscle groups essential for maintaining stability, balance, and mobility as we age. We'll explore the benefits of core and leg exercises for seniors and then dive into a series of seated exercises designed to strengthen these areas safely and effectively.

## Benefits of Core and Leg Exercises for Seniors

Core and leg exercises offer numerous benefits for seniors, including:

- **Improved Stability:** Strengthening the core and leg muscles helps improve balance and stability, reducing the risk of falls and injuries.
- **Enhanced Mobility:** Strong core and leg muscles support better posture and movement, making everyday activities like walking, standing, and bending easier and more comfortable.
- **Prevention of Back Pain:** A strong core can alleviate pressure on the spine and reduce the risk of developing back pain or discomfort.
- **Increased Independence:** By maintaining strength and function in the core and legs, seniors can maintain their independence and continue to engage in activities of daily living with confidence.

Now, let's explore some core and leg exercises that seniors can incorporate into their chair yoga practice.

# Core Exercises

## Seated Cat-Cow Pose

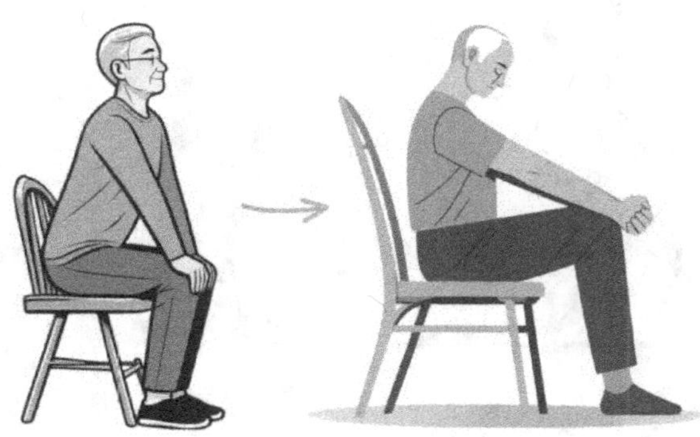

1. Sit tall in your chair with your feet flat on the floor and your hands resting on your thighs.
2. Inhale as you arch your back, lifting your chest and tilting your pelvis forward (Cow Pose).
3. Exhale as you round your spine, tucking your chin towards your chest and drawing your navel in towards your spine (Cat Pose).
4. Continue flowing between Cat and Cow poses, moving with your breath and focusing on articulating each vertebra.
5. Repeat this sequence for several repetitions, allowing your breath to guide your movement and deepen the stretch in your spine.

# Seated Side Plank (with Chair Support)

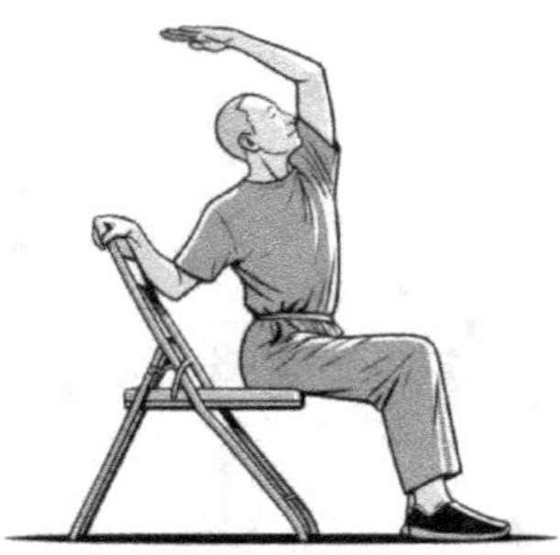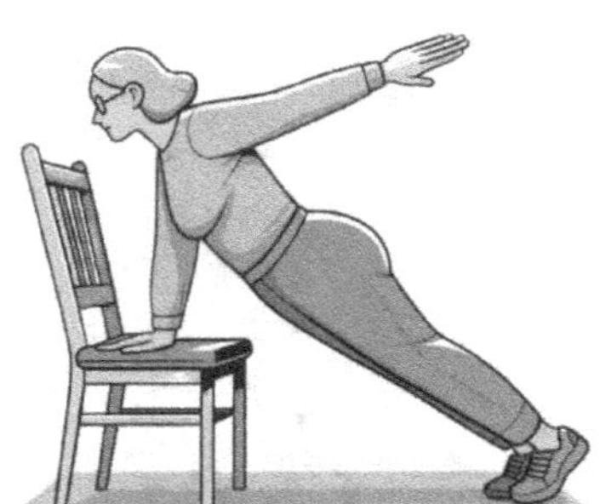

1. Sit sideways on your chair with your right hand placed on the seat and your legs extended to the side.
2. Press down through your right hand and lift your hips off the chair, creating a straight line from your head to your heels.
3. Engage your core muscles to stabilize your body and hold the position for a few breaths.
4. Lower your hips back down to the chair and switch sides, placing your left hand on the seat and repeating the side plank on the opposite side.
5. Continue alternating between right and left side planks for several repetitions, focusing on maintaining proper form and alignment.

# Seated Abdominal Crunches (Modified)

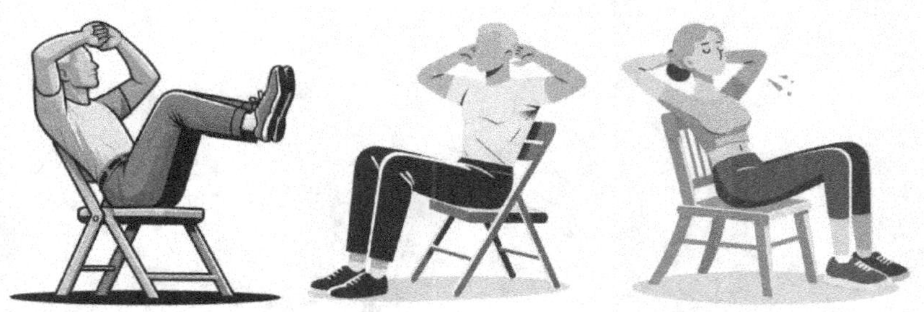

1.  Sit tall in your chair with your feet flat on the floor and your hands behind your head, elbows wide.
2.  Engage your core muscles and exhale as you gently lean back, keeping your spine long and your chest lifted.
3.  Inhale as you return to an upright position, using your abdominal muscles to lift your torso back to center.
4.  Repeat this movement for several repetitions, focusing on using your core muscles to initiate the movement rather than relying on momentum.
5.  For an added challenge, you can cross your arms over your chest or extend your arms straight out in front of you as you perform the crunches.

# Leg Exercises

## Chair Leg Extensions

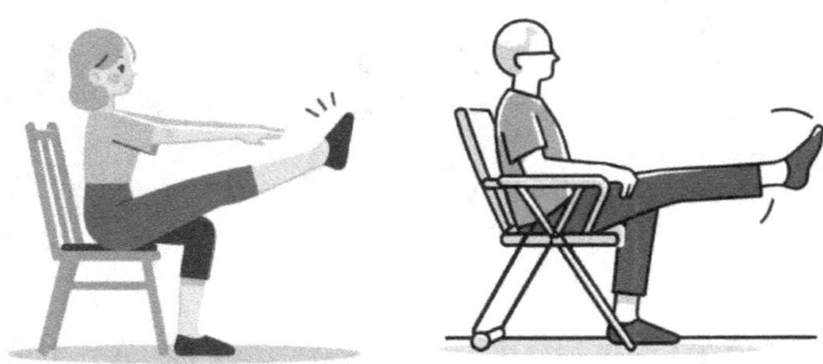

1. Sit tall in your chair with your feet flat on the floor and your hands resting on your thighs.
2. Extend your right leg straight out in front of you, keeping your foot flexed and your knee straight.
3. Hold the extended position for a few breaths, engaging your quadriceps muscles to lift your leg.
4. Lower your right leg back down to the floor and repeat the movement with your left leg.
5. Continue alternating between right and left leg extensions for several repetitions, focusing on maintaining control and stability throughout the movement.

# Seated Knee Extensions

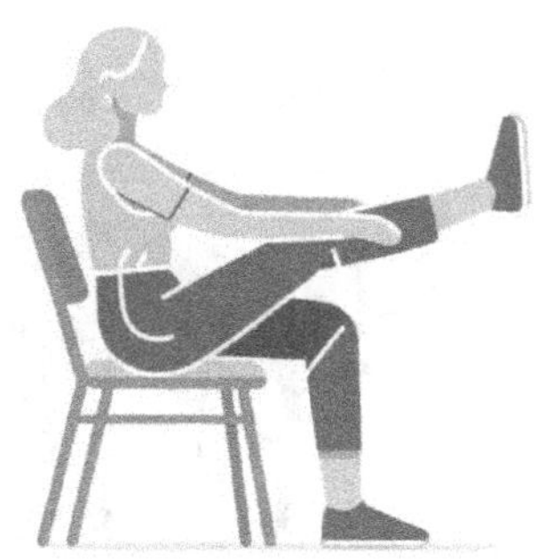 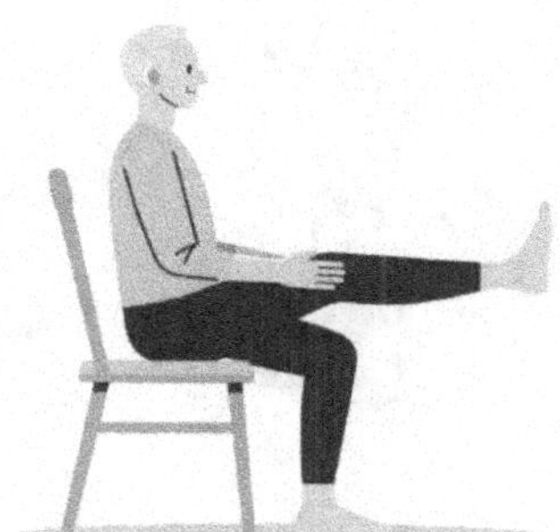

1.  Sit tall in your chair with your feet flat on the floor and your hands resting on your thighs.
2.  Extend your right leg straight out in front of you, lifting your foot slightly off the floor.
3.  Keeping your knee straight, slowly lower your right foot back down to the floor, tapping your toes lightly.
4.  Repeat the knee extension with your right leg for several repetitions, then switch to your left leg.
5.  Continue alternating between right and left knee extensions, moving with control and precision.

## Heel Slides

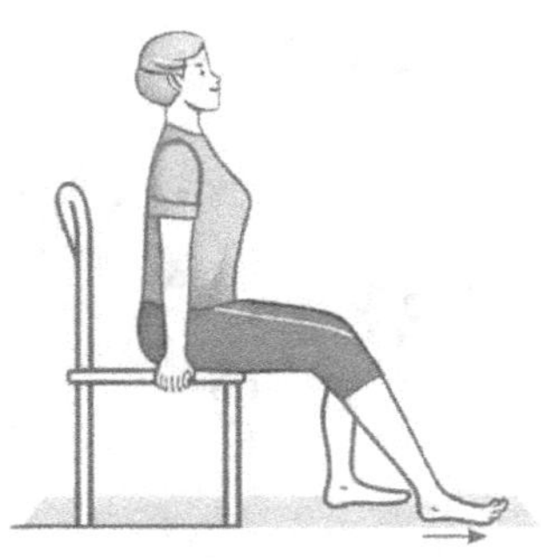 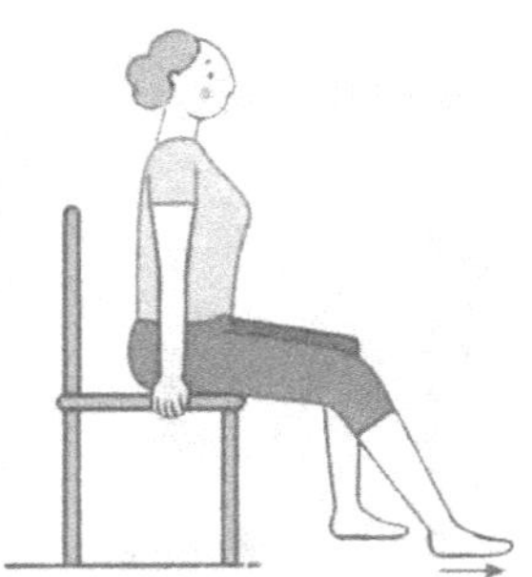

1. Sit comfortably in your chair with your feet flat on the floor and your hands resting on your thighs.
2. Slide your right heel forward along the floor, straightening your leg as much as possible without lifting your foot off the floor.
3. Flex your right foot as you slide it forward, feeling a stretch along the back of your leg.
4. Slowly slide your right heel back to the starting position, returning to a seated position with your knee bent.
5. Repeat the heel slide with your left leg, sliding your left heel forward and then back.
6. Continue alternating between right and left heel slides for several repetitions, focusing on maintaining a smooth and controlled movement.

# Calf Raises

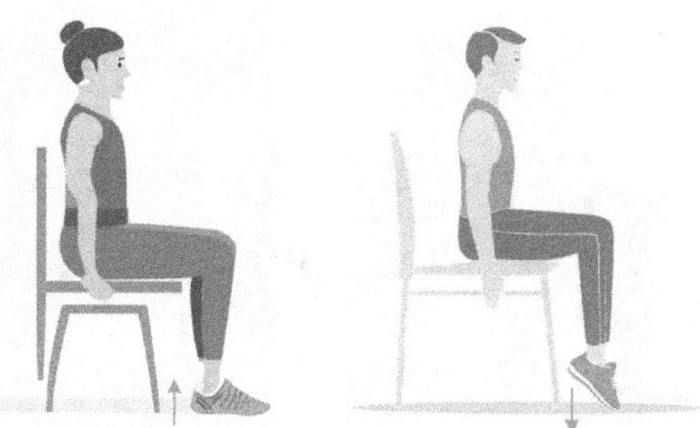

1.  Sit tall in your chair with your feet flat on the floor
    and your hands resting on your thighs.
2.  Press down through the balls of your feet and lift
    your heels off the floor, raising your body up onto
    your toes.
3.  Hold the raised position for a few breaths, feeling the
    contraction in your calf muscles.
4.  Lower your heels back down to the floor, returning
    to a seated position with both feet flat on the floor.
5.  Repeat the calf raises for several repetitions, focusing
    on lifting and lowering with control and precision.

## Inner and Outer Thigh Stretches

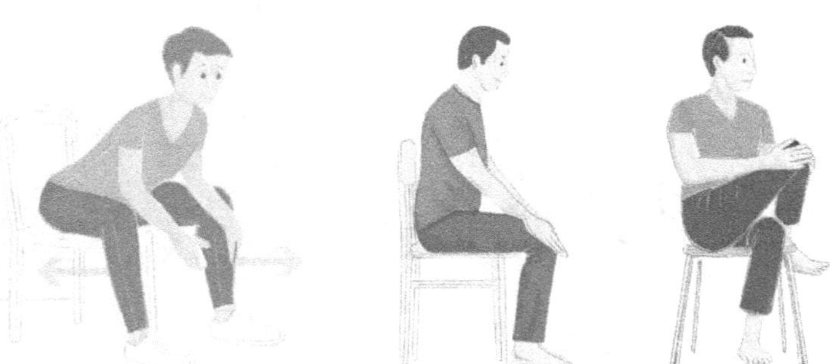

1. Sit tall in your chair with your feet flat on the floor and your hands resting on your thighs.
2. Open your right leg out to the side, keeping your knee bent and your foot flat on the floor.
3. Place your right hand on the inside of your right thigh and gently press your knee towards the floor, feeling a stretch along the inner thigh.
4. Hold the stretch for a few breaths, then switch to the opposite side, stretching your left inner thigh.
5. Next, cross your right ankle over your left knee, flexing your right foot to protect your knee joint.
6. Place your right hand on the outside of your right thigh and gently press your knee away from your body, feeling a stretch along the outer hip and thigh.
7. Hold the stretch for a few breaths, then switch to the opposite side, stretching your left outer thigh.
8. Continue alternating between inner and outer thigh stretches for several repetitions, moving slowly and gently to avoid straining your muscles.

# Conclusion

By incorporating these core and leg exercises into your chair yoga practice, you can build strength, stability, and flexibility in key muscle groups essential for maintaining overall health and well-being. Remember to move mindfully, listening to your body and respecting your limits. With consistent practice, you'll gradually notice improvements in your posture, balance, and mobility, allowing you to enjoy a more active and independent lifestyle as you age. In the following chapters, we'll continue to explore additional exercises and sequences to support your journey towards optimal health and vitality. Keep up the great work!

# Chapter 04

## Improving Upper Body Strength and Flexibility

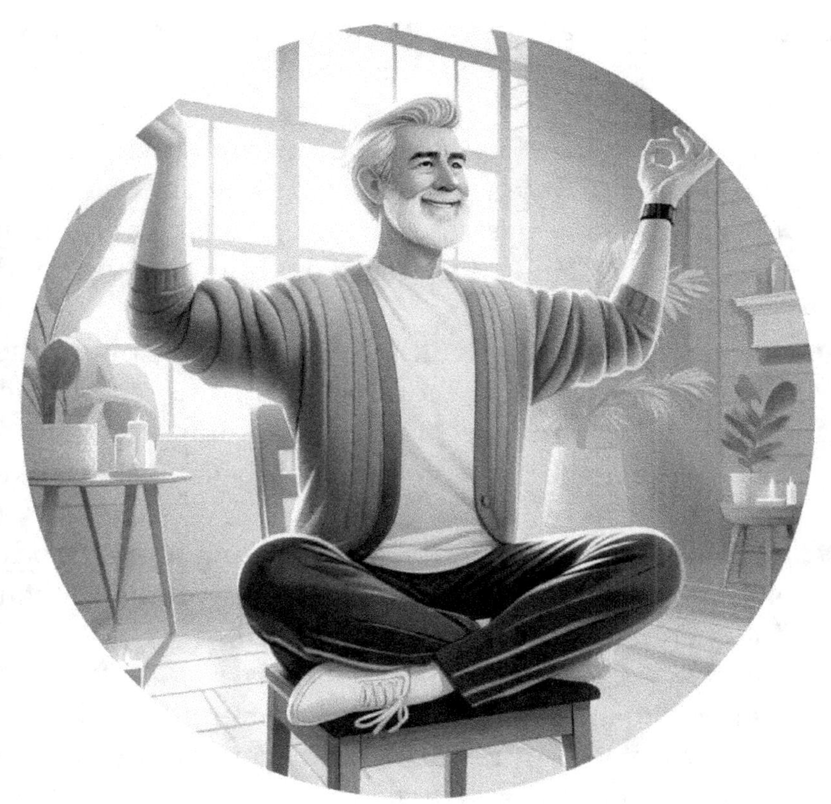

In this chapter, we'll focus on exercises to enhance upper body strength and flexibility, specifically tailored for seniors. We'll explore the benefits of upper body exercises and then delve into a series of seated movements designed to target the shoulders, arms, chest, and back. These exercises will help seniors build muscle strength, improve joint mobility, and maintain overall physical function.

# Benefits of Upper Body Exercises for Seniors

Engaging in regular upper body exercises offers a variety of benefits for seniors, including:

- **Improved Functional Strength:** Strengthening the muscles of the upper body helps seniors perform everyday activities more easily, such as lifting groceries, reaching for items on high shelves, and carrying objects.
- **Enhanced Joint Health:** By strengthening the muscles surrounding the shoulders, arms, chest, and back, seniors can help protect their joints from injury and reduce the risk of developing conditions like arthritis.
- **Increased Independence:** Maintaining upper body strength allows seniors to maintain their independence and continue to perform activities of daily living with confidence and ease.
- **Better Posture and Balance:** Strengthening the muscles of the upper back and shoulders can help improve posture and balance, reducing the risk of falls and promoting overall stability.

Now, let's explore some effective upper body exercises for seniors.

# Shoulders and Arms

## Seated Arm Raises (Lateral and Frontal)

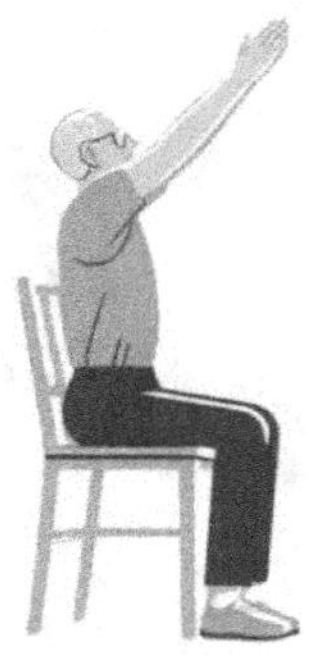 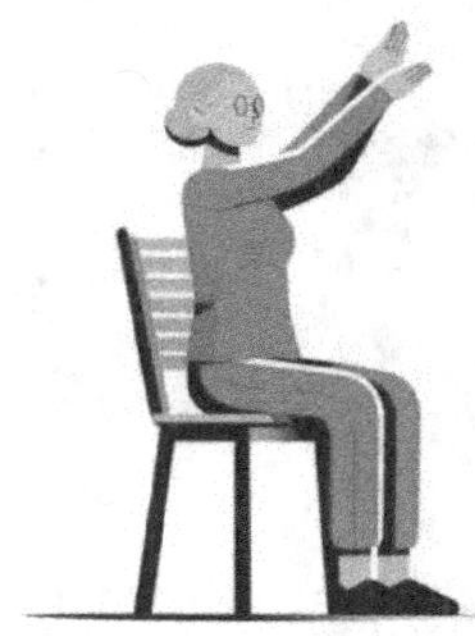

1. Sit tall in your chair with your feet flat on the floor and your arms resting by your sides.
2. Inhale as you raise both arms out to the sides, lifting them up to shoulder height (Lateral Raises).
3. Exhale as you lower your arms back down to your sides, maintaining control and stability throughout the movement.
4. Repeat the lateral raises for several repetitions, focusing on engaging your shoulder muscles and keeping your chest open.
5. Next, inhale as you raise both arms straight out in front of you, lifting them up to shoulder height (Frontal Raises).
6. Exhale as you lower your arms back down to your sides, maintaining a slow and controlled movement.

7.  Repeat the frontal raises for several repetitions, keeping your shoulders relaxed and your core engaged.

## Bicep Curls (Using Water Bottles)

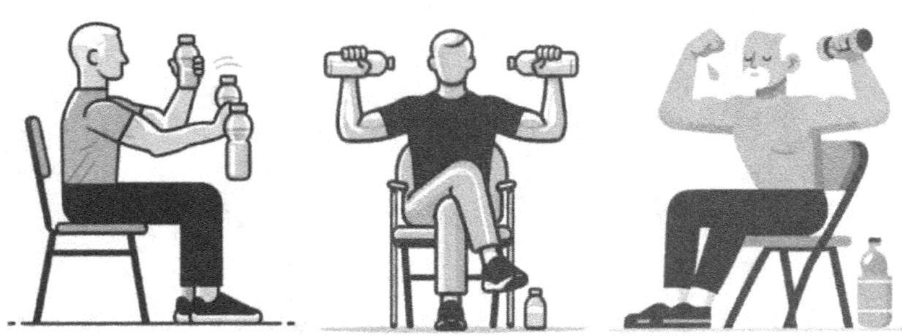

1.  Hold a water bottle in each hand, palms facing forward, and sit tall in your chair with your feet flat on the floor.
2.  Inhale as you bend your elbows, bringing the water bottles up towards your shoulders (Bicep Curls).
3.  Exhale as you lower the water bottles back down to your sides, maintaining control and stability throughout the movement.
4.  Repeat the bicep curls for several repetitions, focusing on squeezing your bicep muscles at the top of the movement.
5.  Keep your wrists straight and your elbows close to your body as you perform the curls, avoiding any swinging or jerking motions.

# Triceps Dips (Using Chair Arms)

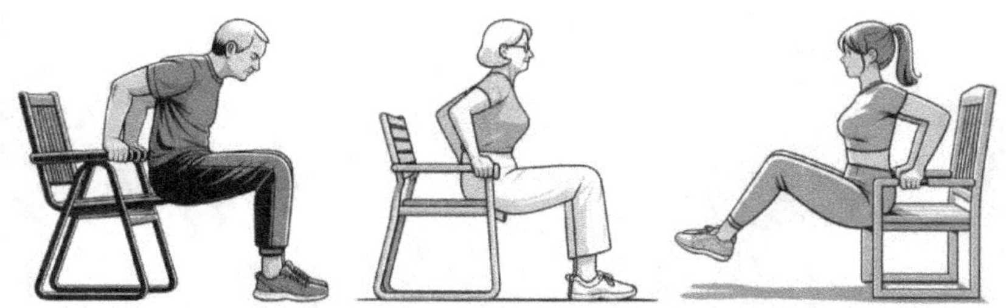

1.  Sit towards the front edge of your chair with your hands gripping the edges of the seat, fingers facing forward.
2.  Inhale as you lift your hips off the chair, straightening your arms and extending your legs out in front of you.
3.  Exhale as you bend your elbows, lowering your hips towards the floor and keeping your back close to the chair.
4.  Inhale to press back up to the starting position, straightening your arms and lifting your hips back up.
5.  Repeat the triceps dips for several repetitions, focusing on engaging your triceps muscles and keeping your core tight.
6.  If this variation is too challenging, you can perform a modified version of triceps dips by keeping your knees bent and your feet flat on the floor.

# Chest and Back

## Seated Chest Openers

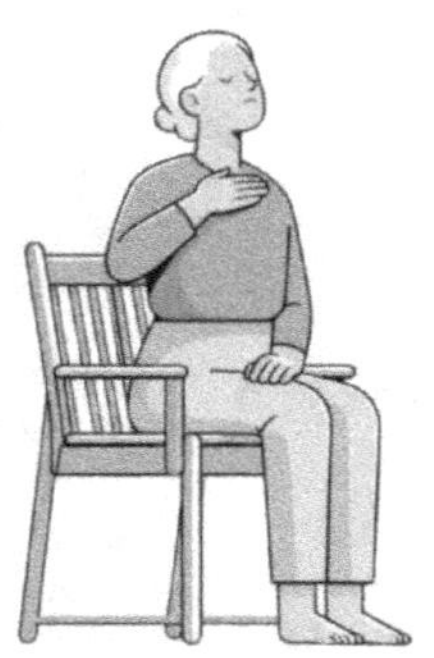 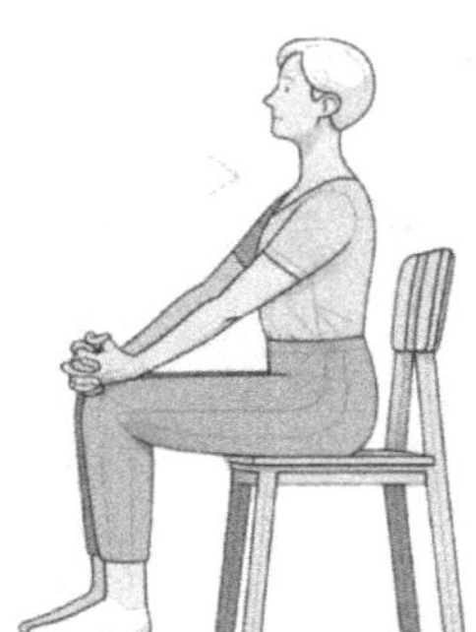

1. Sit tall in your chair with your feet flat on the floor and your hands clasped behind your back.
2. Inhale as you squeeze your shoulder blades together and lift your chest towards the ceiling, opening up your chest and shoulders.
3. Exhale as you release the stretch, bringing your hands back to your sides and relaxing your shoulders.
4. Repeat the chest openers for several repetitions, focusing on expanding your chest and improving posture.
5. You can also perform this stretch by interlacing your fingers behind your back and straightening your arms as you lift your chest.

## Seated Rowing (Using Resistance Bands - Optional)

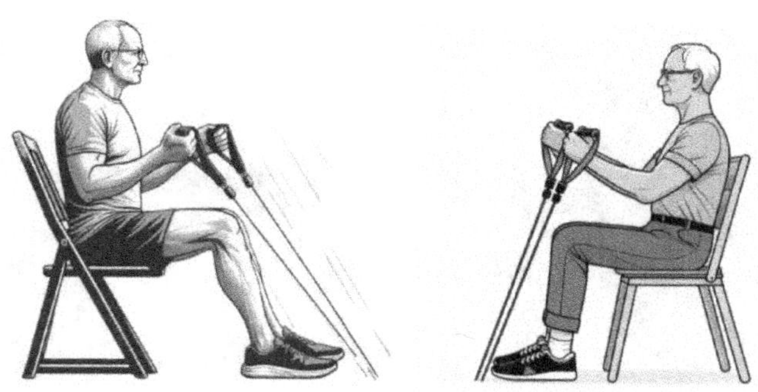

1.  Sit tall in your chair with your feet flat on the floor and a resistance band looped around the bottoms of your feet.
2.  Hold the ends of the resistance band in each hand, palms facing each other, and keep your arms extended in front of you.
3.  Inhale as you bend your elbows and pull the resistance band towards your body, squeezing your shoulder blades together.
4.  Exhale as you slowly release the tension in the resistance band and straighten your arms back out in front of you.
5.  Repeat the rowing motion for several repetitions, focusing on engaging your back muscles and maintaining proper posture.
6.  You can adjust the resistance of the band by gripping it closer to or farther from your feet, depending on your strength and fitness level.

## Seated Spinal Twists

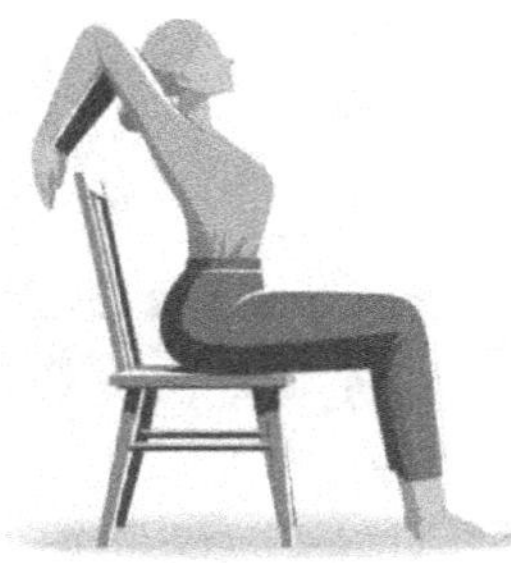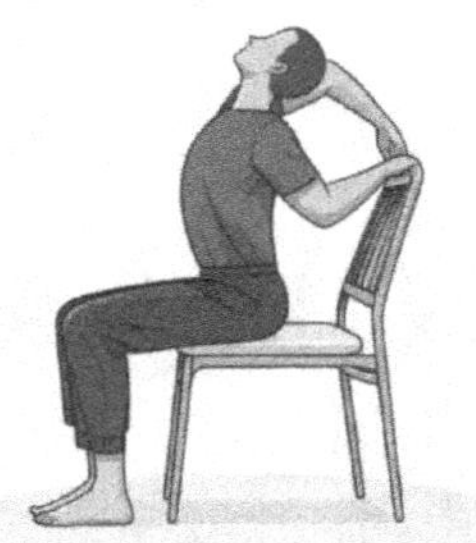

1.  Sit tall in your chair with your feet flat on the floor and your hands resting on your thighs.
2.  Inhale as you lengthen your spine, lifting through the crown of your head.
3.  Exhale as you twist your torso to the right, placing your left hand on the outside of your right thigh and your right hand on the back of the chair.
4.  Inhale to lengthen your spine and deepen the twist, turning your gaze over your right shoulder.
5.  Exhale as you release the twist and return to center.
6.  Repeat the twist to the left side, placing your right hand on the outside of your left thigh and your left hand on the back of the chair.
7.  Inhale to lengthen your spine and deepen the twist, turning your gaze over your left shoulder.
8.  Exhale as you release the twist and return to center.
9.  Continue alternating between right and left spinal twists for several repetitions, moving with your breath and maintaining a smooth, controlled movement.

# Conclusion

By incorporating these upper body exercises into your chair yoga practice, you can strengthen and tone the muscles of your shoulders, arms, chest, and back, promoting overall strength and flexibility. Remember to move mindfully, listening to your body and respecting your limits. With consistent practice, you'll gradually notice improvements in your posture, range of motion, and functional strength, allowing you to enjoy a more active and independent lifestyle as you age. In the following chapters, we'll continue to explore additional exercises and sequences to support your journey towards optimal health and vitality. Keep up the great work!

# Chapter 05

## Chair Yoga for Balance and Coordination

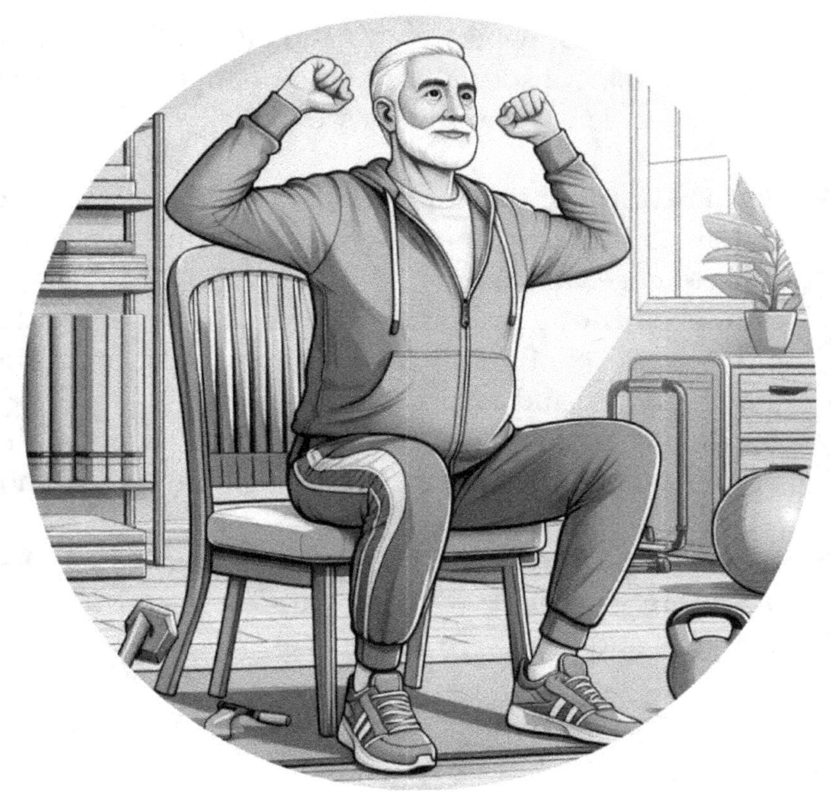

In this chapter, we'll explore chair yoga poses and exercises specifically designed to improve balance and coordination for seniors. We'll discuss the importance and benefits of balance training for older adults and then dive into a series of seated and standing poses that target key muscle groups involved in maintaining stability and coordination.

# Importance and Benefits of Balance for Seniors

Balance is a crucial aspect of functional movement and overall well-being, especially for seniors. Here are some reasons why balance training is essential:

- **Fall Prevention:** Improving balance reduces the risk of falls and related injuries, which can have serious consequences for seniors.
- **Enhanced Mobility:** Better balance allows seniors to move more confidently and efficiently, supporting independence and quality of life.
- **Improved Posture:** Balance training helps maintain proper posture, reducing strain on the muscles and joints.
- **Increased Confidence:** As balance improves, seniors feel more confident in their ability to perform daily activities and engage in physical exercise.

Now, let's explore some chair yoga poses and exercises to enhance balance and coordination.

# Chair Yoga Poses for Balance and Coordination

## Mountain Pose

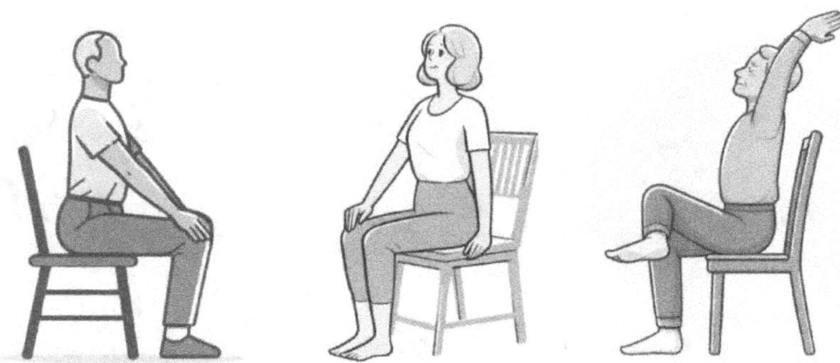

1.  Sit tall in your chair with your feet flat on the floor and your hands resting on your thighs.
2.  Ground down through your feet and imagine roots growing from the soles of your feet into the earth.
3.  Lengthen through your spine, lifting through the crown of your head, and roll your shoulders back and down.
4.  Engage your core muscles to support your spine and maintain a strong, stable posture.
5.  Take several deep breaths in this Mountain Pose, feeling grounded and centered.

## Tree Pose

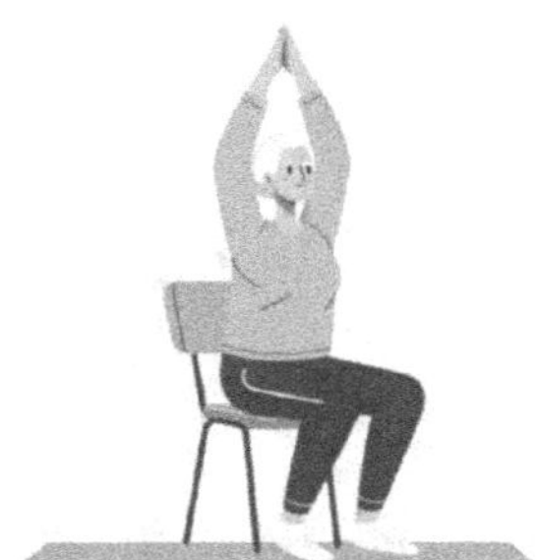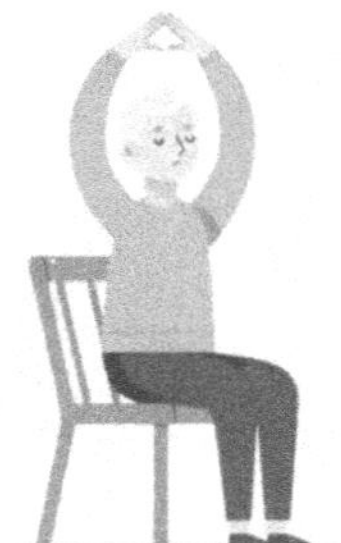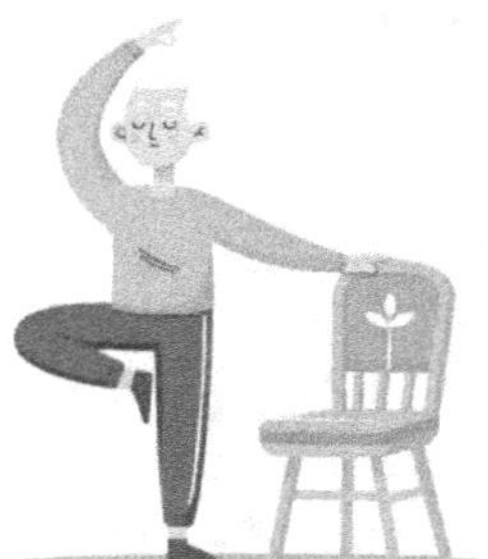

1.  Sit tall in your chair with your feet flat on the floor and your hands resting on your thighs.
2.  Shift your weight into your left foot and root down through your left leg.
3.  Bend your right knee and place the sole of your right foot on the inner thigh or calf of your left leg, avoiding the knee joint.
4.  Press your right foot into your left leg and engage your core for balance.
5.  Bring your palms together at your heart center or extend your arms overhead like branches of a tree.
6.  Hold the Tree Pose for several breaths, then release and switch sides.

## Warrior Pose

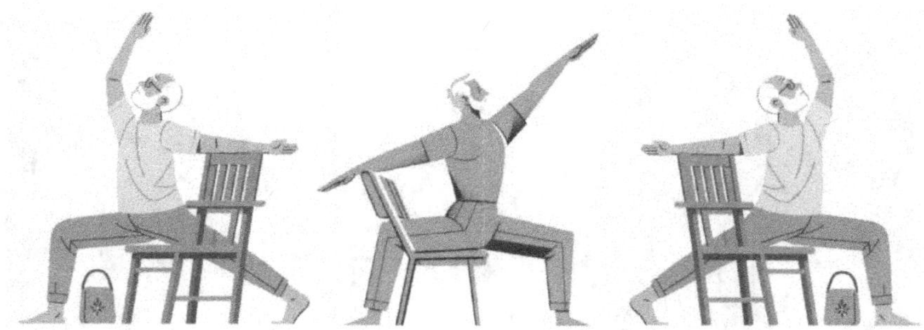

1.  Sit tall in your chair with your feet flat on the floor and your hands resting on your thighs.

2.  Step your right foot back behind you, keeping your toes pointing forward and your heel lifted off the floor.

3.  Bend your left knee to create a 90-degree angle, stacking it directly over your left ankle.

4.  Square your hips towards the front of the chair and reach your arms overhead, lifting through your fingertips.

5.  Engage your core and press firmly into your feet to create a strong, stable base.

6.  Hold the Warrior Pose for several breaths, then switch sides.

## Heel-Toe Pose

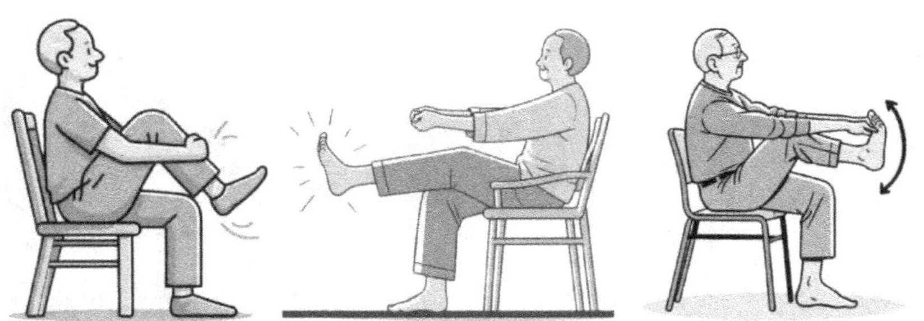

1.  Sit tall in your chair with your feet hip-width apart and your hands resting on your thighs.
2.  Lift your right heel off the floor and place it directly in front of your left toes, creating a straight line with your feet.
3.  Maintain a slight bend in your knees and engage your core muscles for stability.
4.  Hold the Heel-Toe Pose for several breaths, feeling the muscles in your feet and ankles working to maintain balance.
5.  Return to the starting position and repeat the pose on the opposite side.

# Seated Single Leg Raises

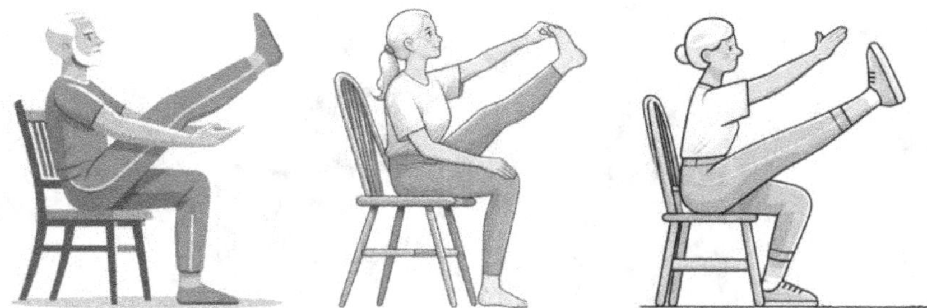

1.  Sit tall in your chair with your feet flat on the floor
    and your hands resting on your thighs.
2.  Extend your right leg out in front of you, lifting it off
    the floor and keeping it straight.
3.  Hold the raised position for a few breaths, engaging
    your core and maintaining stability.
4.  Lower your right leg back down to the floor and
    repeat the movement with your left leg.
5.  Continue alternating between right and left single
    leg raises for several repetitions, focusing on control
    and balance.

## Heel-Toe Rock

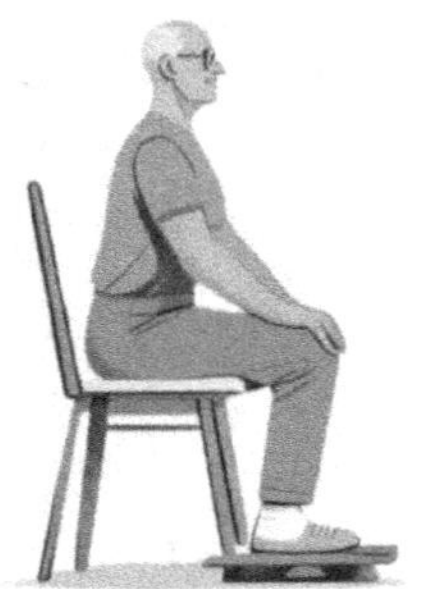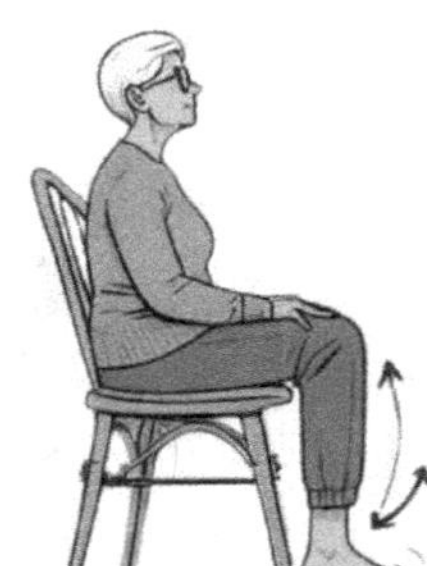

1.  Sit tall in your chair with your feet hip-width apart and your hands resting on your thighs.
2.  Shift your weight onto your heels, lifting your toes off the floor and keeping your heels grounded.
3.  Hold the position for a few breaths, feeling the stretch in the bottoms of your feet and ankles.
4.  Shift your weight forward onto your toes, lifting your heels off the floor and keeping your toes grounded.
5.  Hold the position for a few breaths, feeling the stretch in your calves and ankles.
6.  Continue rocking back and forth between heels and toes, moving with your breath and maintaining balance.

# Seated Figure Eights (with Arms)

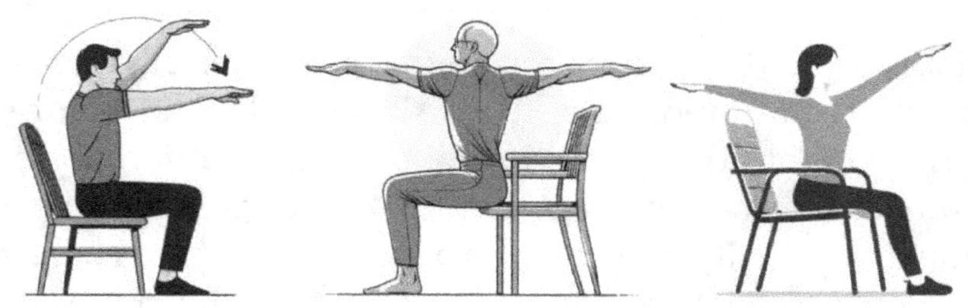

1. Sit tall in your chair with your feet flat on the floor and your hands resting on your thighs.
2. Extend your arms out to the sides at shoulder height, palms facing down.
3. Inhale as you draw a figure eight shape with your right hand, moving it across your body towards the left.
4. Exhale as you continue the figure eight shape, moving your right hand back across your body towards the right.
5. Repeat this movement for several repetitions, focusing on smooth, controlled motions and maintaining stability in your torso.
6. After completing repetitions with your right hand, switch to your left hand and repeat the figure eight motion.
7. Continue alternating between right and left figure eights for several repetitions, moving with your breath and staying focused on coordination and balance.

# Conclusion

By incorporating these chair yoga poses and exercises into your daily routine, you can improve balance, stability, and coordination, enhancing overall physical function and reducing the risk of falls and injuries. Remember to move mindfully, paying attention to your body and respecting your limits. With consistent practice, you'll gradually notice improvements in your balance and coordination, allowing you to move with confidence and ease. In the following chapters, we'll continue to explore additional exercises and sequences to support your journey towards optimal health and vitality. Keep up the great work!

# Chapter 06

# Increasing Flexibility Throughout the Body

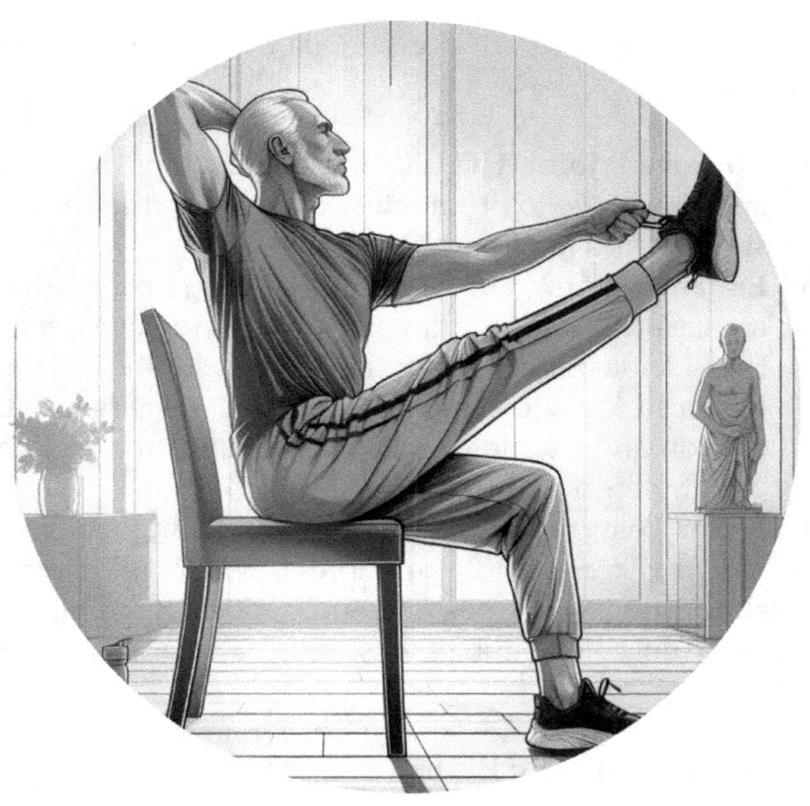

In this chapter, we'll explore a variety of chair yoga exercises and stretches aimed at increasing flexibility throughout the body, specifically tailored for seniors. We'll discuss the benefits of flexibility training and then delve into a series of seated stretches designed to target different muscle groups and improve overall range of motion.

# Benefits of Flexibility Exercises for Seniors

Flexibility exercises offer numerous benefits for seniors, including:

- **Improved Joint Health:** Stretching helps maintain and improve joint mobility, reducing the risk of stiffness and joint pain.
- **Enhanced Range of Motion:** Regular stretching can increase flexibility, allowing seniors to move more freely and comfortably in their daily activities.
- **Reduced Muscle Tension:** Stretching releases muscle tension and promotes relaxation, alleviating feelings of tightness and discomfort.
- **Better Posture and Alignment:** Stretching elongates the muscles and promotes better alignment, supporting good posture and reducing the risk of musculoskeletal imbalances.

Now, let's explore some chair yoga stretches to promote flexibility throughout the body.

# Chair Yoga Stretches for Flexibility

## Gentle Seated Forward Bends with Variations

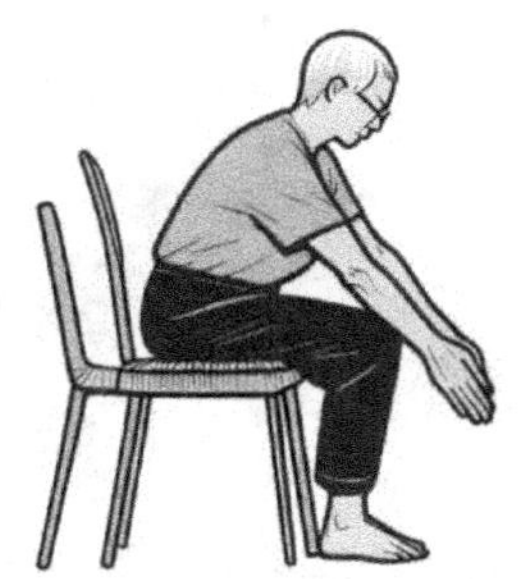 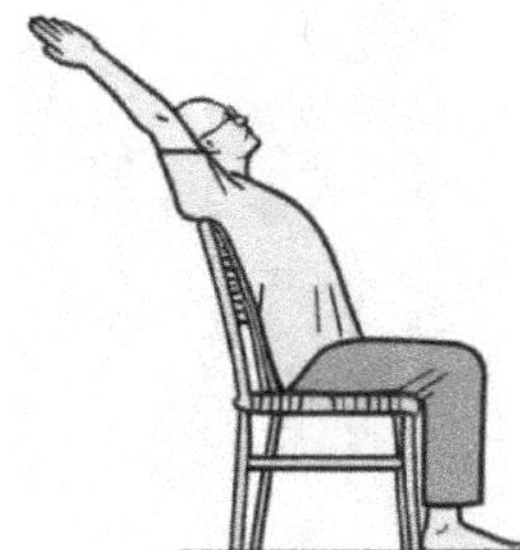

1. Sit tall in your chair with your feet flat on the floor and your hands resting on your thighs.
2. Inhale as you lengthen through your spine, lifting through the crown of your head.
3. Exhale as you hinge forward from your hips, leading with your chest and reaching your hands towards your feet.
4. Hold the forward bend for several breaths, feeling a gentle stretch along the back of your legs and spine.
5. Variation 1: Place your hands on your shins or ankles for support if you cannot reach your feet comfortably.
6. Variation 2: Hold onto the sides of your chair seat and gently press your chest towards your thighs to deepen the stretch.
7. Variation 3: Interlace your fingers behind your back and extend your arms overhead, lifting your chest and opening your shoulders as you fold forward.

## Seated Side Stretches (Arms Reaching Overhead)

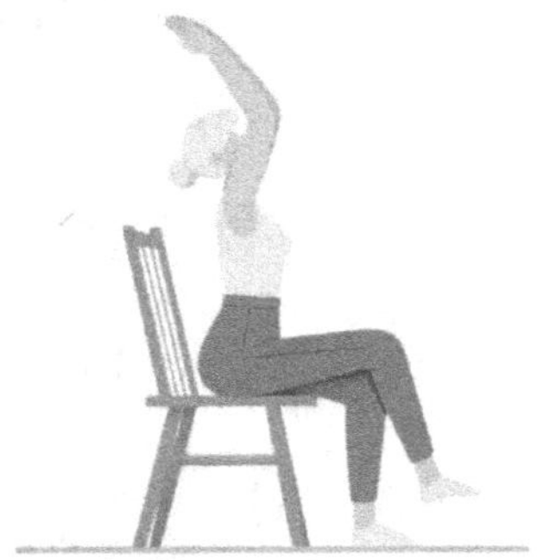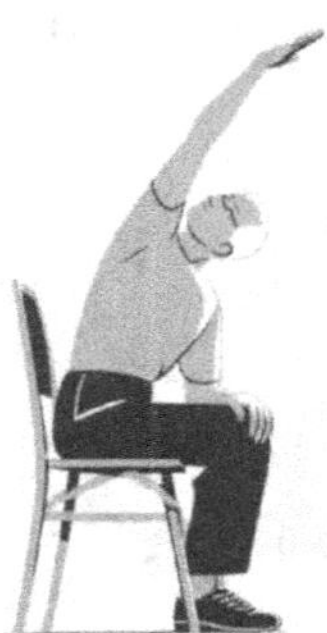

1. Sit tall in your chair with your feet flat on the floor and your hands resting on your thighs.
2. Inhale as you reach your right arm overhead, stretching up towards the ceiling.
3. Exhale as you lean to the left, stretching the right side of your body.
4. Hold the side stretch for several breaths, feeling a deep stretch along the right side of your torso and arm.
5. Inhale to return to the center and switch sides, reaching your left arm overhead and leaning to the right.
6. Continue alternating between right and left side stretches, moving with your breath and maintaining length through your spine.

## Seated Hamstring Stretch (Using a Strap - Optional)

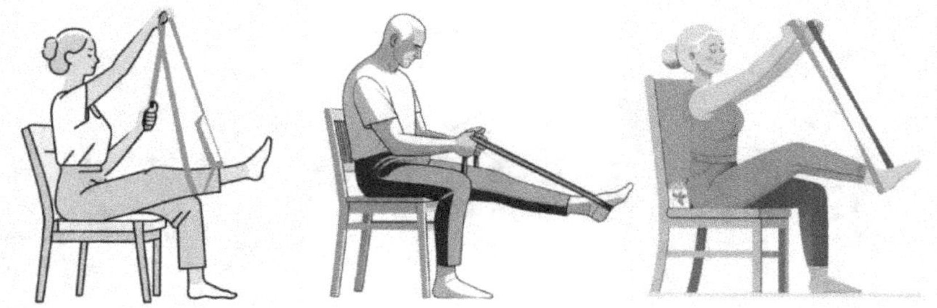

1. Sit tall in your chair with your legs extended straight out in front of you and your feet flexed.
2. Loop a yoga strap or towel around the bottom of your right foot and hold one end of the strap in each hand.
3. Inhale as you lengthen through your spine, lifting your chest.
4. Exhale as you gently hinge forward from your hips, keeping your back flat and your shoulders relaxed.
5. Hold the stretch for several breaths, feeling a deep stretch along the back of your right leg.
6. Inhale to return to an upright position and switch sides, stretching the left hamstring.
7. Continue alternating between right and left hamstring stretches, moving with your breath and maintaining a gentle, steady stretch.

# Seated Neck Stretches (Lateral and Rotational)

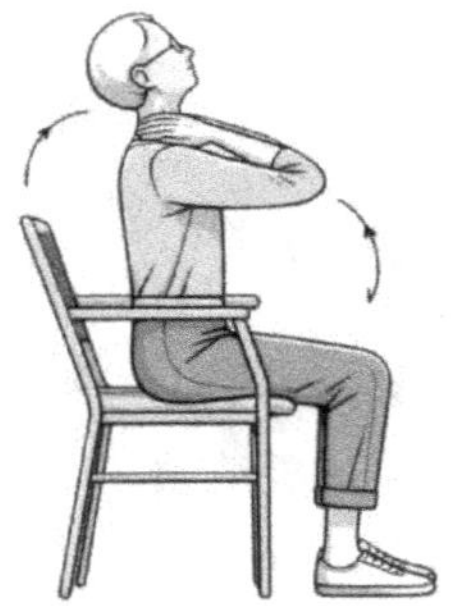 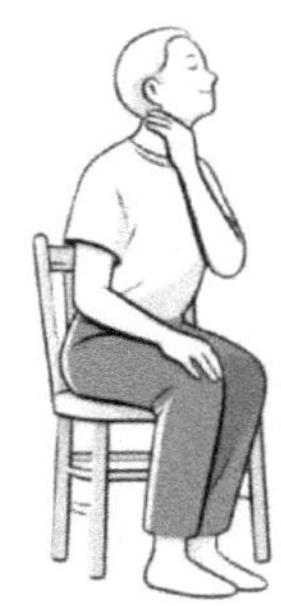 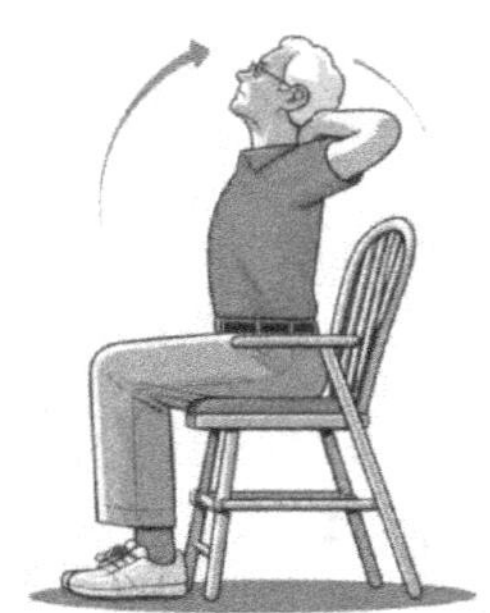

1.  Sit tall in your chair with your feet flat on the floor and your hands resting on your thighs.
2.  Inhale as you lengthen through your spine, lifting your chest and relaxing your shoulders.
3.  Exhale as you tilt your head to the right, bringing your right ear towards your right shoulder.
4.  Hold the stretch for several breaths, feeling a gentle stretch along the left side of your neck.
5.  Inhale to return to the center and exhale as you tilt your head to the left, bringing your left ear towards your left shoulder.
6.  Continue alternating between right and left neck stretches, moving with your breath and maintaining a relaxed, steady stretch.
7.  For a rotational neck stretch, inhale as you lengthen through your spine and exhale as you gently rotate your head to the right, looking over your right shoulder. Hold for a few breaths and then repeat on the left side.

# Cat-Cow Pose

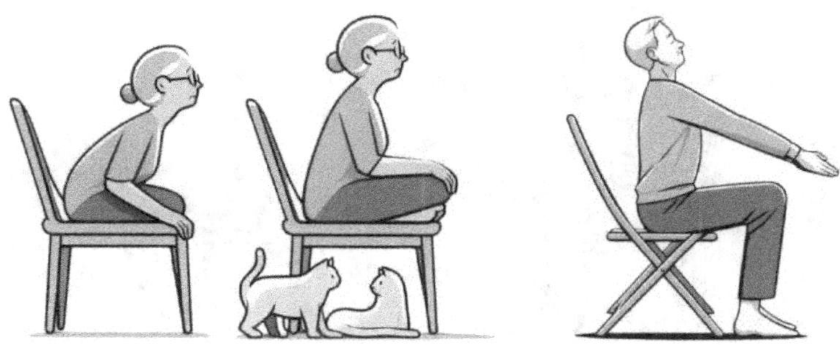

1.  Sit tall in your chair with your feet flat on the floor and your hands resting on your thighs.

2.  Inhale as you arch your back, lifting your chest and tilting your pelvis forward (Cow Pose).

3.  Exhale as you round your spine, tucking your chin towards your chest and drawing your navel in towards your spine (Cat Pose).

4.  Continue flowing between Cat and Cow poses, moving with your breath and focusing on articulating each vertebra.

5.  Repeat this sequence for several repetitions, allowing your breath to guide your movement and deepen the stretch in your spine.

**Eagle Arm**

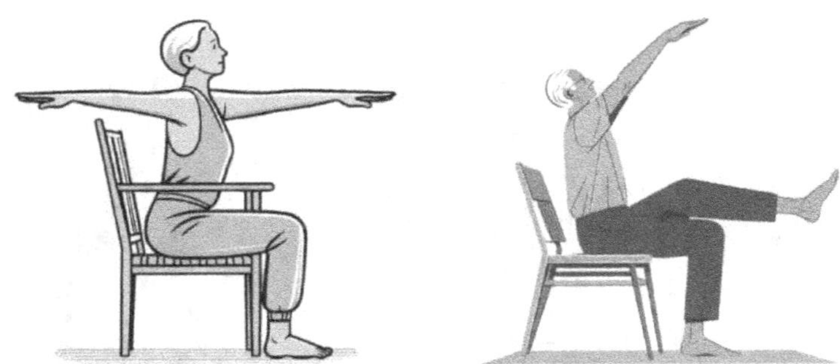

1.  Sit tall in your chair with your feet flat on the floor and your hands resting on your thighs.
2.  Inhale as you reach your arms out to the sides at shoulder height, palms facing down.
3.  Exhale as you cross your right arm over your left arm, bringing your palms together if possible.
4.  Inhale to lift your elbows slightly, feeling a stretch between your shoulder blades.
5.  Hold the Eagle Arm stretch for several breaths, then release and switch sides, crossing your left arm over your right.
6.  Continue alternating between right and left Eagle Arm stretches, focusing on keeping your shoulders relaxed and your breath steady.

# Conclusion

Incorporating these chair yoga stretches into your daily routine can help increase flexibility throughout your body, promoting better joint mobility, muscle relaxation, and overall well-being. Remember to move mindfully and listen to your body, respecting your limits and avoiding any pain or discomfort. With consistent practice, you'll gradually notice improvements in your flexibility and range of motion, allowing you to move with greater ease and comfort in your daily activities. In the following chapters, we'll continue to explore additional exercises and sequences to support your journey towards optimal health and vitality. Keep up the great work!

# Chapter 07

## The Ultimate 28-Day Chair Yoga Plan

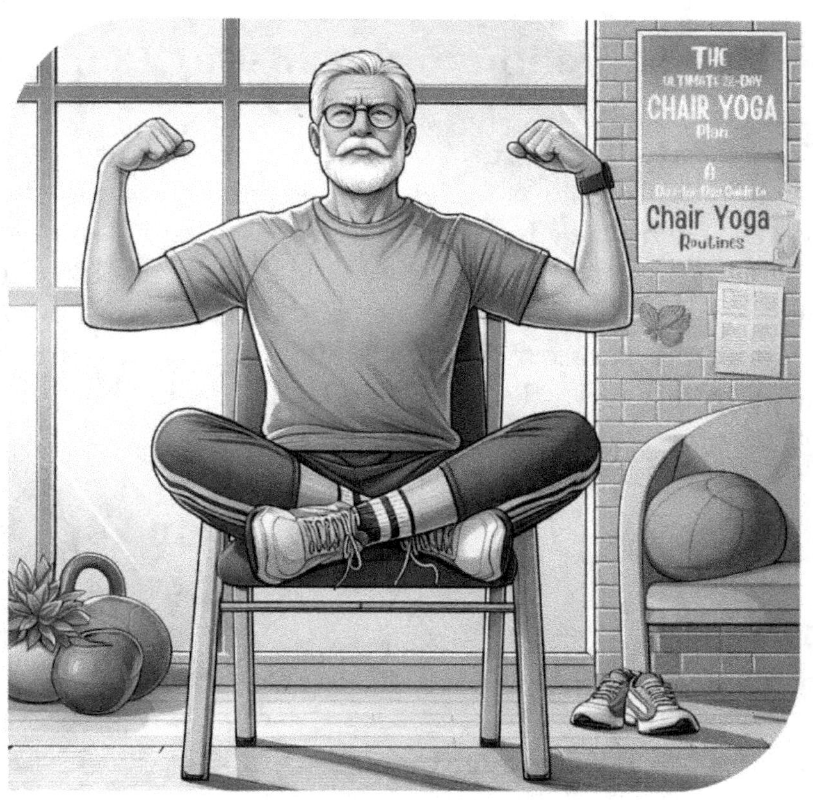

Welcome to the Ultimate 28-Day Chair Yoga Plan! This comprehensive program is designed to help seniors over 60 improve their strength, flexibility, balance, and overall well-being through a series of gentle chair yoga exercises. Each day's routine is carefully crafted to target all major muscle groups and provide a balanced workout in just 10-15 minutes. Whether you're new to yoga or have been practicing for years, this plan offers something for everyone, with modifications provided to accommodate different fitness levels. Let's dive into the details of the plan!

# Introduction to the 28-Day Plan

The 28-Day Chair Yoga Plan is structured to provide a gradual progression of exercises over the course of four weeks. Each week introduces new poses and variations to keep the practice fresh and challenging. The plan begins with foundational poses and gradually builds up to more advanced movements, allowing participants to develop strength, flexibility, and balance at their own pace.

# A Day-by-Day Guide to Chair Yoga Routines

## Week 1: Foundation Building

### Day 1: Gentle Introduction

- **Warm-up:** Neck Rolls, Shoulder Rolls, Deep Breathing (3-5 minutes)

- **Focus Exercises:** Seated Cat-Cow, Seated Arm Raises, Seated Forward Bend (5-7 minutes)
- **Cool-down:** Deep Breathing, Seated Relaxation (2-3 minutes)

## Day 2: Core Strengthening

- **Warm-up:** Neck Rolls, Shoulder Rolls, Deep Breathing (3-5 minutes)
- **Focus Exercises:** Seated Cat-Cow, Seated Side Plank, Seated Abdominal Crunches (5-7 minutes)
- **Cool-down:** Deep Breathing, Seated Relaxation (2-3 minutes)

## Day 3: Balance and Coordination

- **Warm-up:** Neck Rolls, Shoulder Rolls, Deep Breathing (3-5 minutes)
- **Focus Exercises:** Tree Pose, Warrior Pose, Heel-Toe Pose (5-7 minutes)
- **Cool-down:** Deep Breathing, Seated Relaxation (2-3 minutes)

## Day 4: Upper Body Strength

- **Warm-up:** Neck Rolls, Shoulder Rolls, Deep Breathing (3-5 minutes)
- **Focus Exercises:** Seated Arm Raises, Bicep Curls, Triceps Dips (5-7 minutes)
- **Cool-down:** Deep Breathing, Seated Relaxation (2-3 minutes)

## Day 5: Flexibility and Stretching

- **Warm-up:** Neck Rolls, Shoulder Rolls, Deep Breathing (3-5 minutes)
- **Focus Exercises:** Seated Forward Bends, Seated Side Stretches, Seated Hamstring Stretch (5-7 minutes)
- **Cool-down:** Deep Breathing, Seated Relaxation (2-3 minutes)

## Day 6: Rest and Recovery

- Take a break from structured exercise.
- Engage in gentle activities like walking, stretching, or meditation.

## Day 7: Review and Reflection

- Reflect on your progress during the first week.
- Set intentions and goals for the upcoming week.

# Week 2: Progression and Variation

## Day 8: Core and Balance

- **Warm-up:** Neck Rolls, Shoulder Rolls, Deep Breathing (3-5 minutes)
- **Focus Exercises:** Seated Cat-Cow, Seated Side Plank, Tree Pose (5-7 minutes)
- **Cool-down:** Deep Breathing, Seated Relaxation (2-3 minutes)

## Day 9: Lower Body Strength

- **Warm-up:** Neck Rolls, Shoulder Rolls, Deep Breathing (3-5 minutes)
- **Focus Exercises:** Chair Leg Extensions, Seated Knee Extensions, Heel Slides (5-7 minutes)
- **Cool-down:** Deep Breathing, Seated Relaxation (2-3 minutes)

## Day 10: Upper Body Flexibility

- **Warm-up:** Neck Rolls, Shoulder Rolls, Deep Breathing (3-5 minutes)
- **Focus Exercises:** Seated Chest Openers, Seated Rowing, Seated Neck Stretches (5-7 minutes)
- **Cool-down:** Deep Breathing, Seated Relaxation (2-3 minutes)

## Day 11: Balance and Coordination

- **Warm-up:** Neck Rolls, Shoulder Rolls, Deep Breathing (3-5 minutes)
- **Focus Exercises:** Mountain Pose, Seated Single Leg

Raises, Heel-Toe Rock (5-7 minutes)

- **Cool-down:** Deep Breathing, Seated Relaxation (2-3 minutes)

## Day 12: Full Body Stretch

- **Warm-up:** Neck Rolls, Shoulder Rolls, Deep Breathing (3-5 minutes)
- **Focus Exercises:** Seated Forward Bends, Seated Side Stretches, Seated Figure Eights (5-7 minutes)
- **Cool-down:** Deep Breathing, Seated Relaxation (2-3 minutes)

## Day 13: Rest and Recovery

- **Rest and Recovery:** Take a break from structured exercise.
- **Engage in Gentle Activities:** Practice gentle stretching, walking, or meditation to support recovery and relaxation.

## Day 14: Review and Reflection

- **Reflect on Progress:** Review your experiences and progress during the first week of the program.
- **Set Intentions:** Set intentions and goals for the upcoming week, focusing on areas you'd like to improve or explore further.

# Week 3: Strength and Stability

## Day 15: Core and Balance

- **Warm-up:** Neck Rolls, Shoulder Rolls, Deep Breathing (3-5 minutes)
- **Focus Exercises:** Seated Cat-Cow, Seated Side Plank, Tree Pose (5-7 minutes)
- **Cool-down:** Deep Breathing, Seated Relaxation (2-3 minutes)

## Day 16: Lower Body Strength

- **Warm-up:** Neck Rolls, Shoulder Rolls, Deep Breathing (3-5 minutes)
- **Focus Exercises:** Chair Leg Extensions, Seated Knee Extensions, Heel Slides (5-7 minutes)
- **Cool-down:** Deep Breathing, Seated Relaxation (2-3 minutes)

## Day 17: Upper Body Flexibility

- **Warm-up:** Neck Rolls, Shoulder Rolls, Deep Breathing (3-5 minutes)
- **Focus Exercises:** Seated Chest Openers, Seated Rowing, Seated Neck Stretches (5-7 minutes)
- **Cool-down:** Deep Breathing, Seated Relaxation (2-3 minutes)

## Day 18: Balance and Coordination

- **Warm-up:** Neck Rolls, Shoulder Rolls, Deep Breathing (3-5 minutes)
- **Focus Exercises:** Mountain Pose, Seated Single Leg

Raises, Heel-Toe Rock (5-7 minutes)

- **Cool-down:** Deep Breathing, Seated Relaxation (2-3 minutes)

## Day 19: Full Body Stretch

- **Warm-up:** Neck Rolls, Shoulder Rolls, Deep Breathing (3-5 minutes)
- **Focus Exercises:** Seated Forward Bends, Seated Side Stretches, Seated Figure Eights (5-7 minutes)
- **Cool-down:** Deep Breathing, Seated Relaxation (2-3 minutes)

## Day 20: Rest and Recovery

- **Rest and Recovery:** Take a break from structured exercise.
- **Engage in Gentle Activities:** Practice gentle stretching, walking, or meditation to support recovery and relaxation.

## Day 21: Review and Reflection

- **Reflect on Progress:** Review your experiences and progress during the second week of the program.
- **Set Intentions:** Set intentions and goals for the upcoming week, focusing on areas you'd like to improve or explore further.

# Week 4: Integration and Mastery

## Day 22: Advanced Flexibility

- **Warm-up:** Neck Rolls, Shoulder Rolls, Deep Breathing (3-5 minutes)
- **Focus Exercises:** Seated Forward Bends with Advanced Variations, Seated Side Stretches with Extended Holds, Seated Figure Eights with Increased Range of Motion (5-7 minutes)
- **Cool-down:** Deep Breathing, Seated Relaxation (2-3 minutes)

## Day 23: Enhanced Strength

- **Warm-up:** Neck Rolls, Shoulder Rolls, Deep Breathing (3-5 minutes)
- **Focus Exercises:** Seated Arm Raises with Light Weights, Bicep Curls with Increased Resistance, Triceps Dips with Extended Hold (5-7 minutes)
- **Cool-down:** Deep Breathing, Seated Relaxation (2-3 minutes)

## Day 24: Advanced Balance

- **Warm-up:** Neck Rolls, Shoulder Rolls, Deep Breathing (3-5 minutes)
- **Focus Exercises:** Tree Pose with Eyes Closed, Warrior Pose with Extended Hold, Heel-Toe Pose with Added Challenge (5-7 minutes)
- **Cool-down:** Deep Breathing, Seated Relaxation (2-3 minutes)

## Day 25: Mastery of Coordination

- **Warm-up:** Neck Rolls, Shoulder Rolls, Deep Breathing (3-5 minutes)
- **Focus Exercises:** Mountain Pose with Dynamic Arm Movements, Seated Single Leg Raises with Increased Speed, Heel-Toe Rock with Side Reaches (5-7 minutes)
- **Cool-down:** Deep Breathing, Seated Relaxation (2-3 minutes)

## Day 26: Integration of Strength and Flexibility

- **Warm-up:** Neck Rolls, Shoulder Rolls, Deep Breathing (3-5 minutes)
- **Focus Exercises:** Combined Flow of Seated Forward Bends and Seated Chest Openers, Dynamic Arm Stretches, Seated Twists with Added Resistance (5-7 minutes)
- **Cool-down:** Deep Breathing, Seated Relaxation (2-3 minutes)

## Day 27: Mindful Movement

- **Warm-up:** Neck Rolls, Shoulder Rolls, Deep Breathing (3-5 minutes)
- **Focus Exercises:** Mindful Sun Salutations, Slow and Controlled Movements with Breath Awareness, Seated Meditation (5-7 minutes)
- **Cool-down:** Deep Breathing, Seated Relaxation (2-3 minutes)

## Day 28: Celebration and Reflection

- **Celebrate Achievement:** Acknowledge and celebrate

your progress throughout the 28-day program.

- **Reflect on Journey:** Reflect on your experiences, challenges, and achievements, and set intentions for future practice.

Congratulations on completing the Ultimate 28-Day Chair Yoga Plan! May your journey towards greater strength, flexibility, balance, and well-being continue to inspire and uplift you.

# Modifications for Different Fitness Levels

Beginner Modifications: Reduce the intensity and duration of poses, use additional support such as cushions or blocks, and focus on maintaining proper alignment and form.

Intermediate Modifications: Gradually increase the intensity and duration of poses, explore deeper variations of poses, and challenge balance and stability.

Advanced Modifications: Incorporate more challenging variations of poses, experiment with transitions between poses, and focus on refining alignment and breath control.

# Conclusion

The Ultimate 28-Day Chair Yoga Plan offers a structured and progressive approach to improving strength, flexibility, balance, and overall well-being for seniors over 60. By following this comprehensive program, participants can develop a sustainable yoga practice that supports their physical and mental health goals. Remember to listen to your body, honor your limits, and approach each practice with curiosity and compassion. Enjoy your journey towards greater health and vitality!

# Chapter 08

## Staying Motivated and Overcoming Challenges

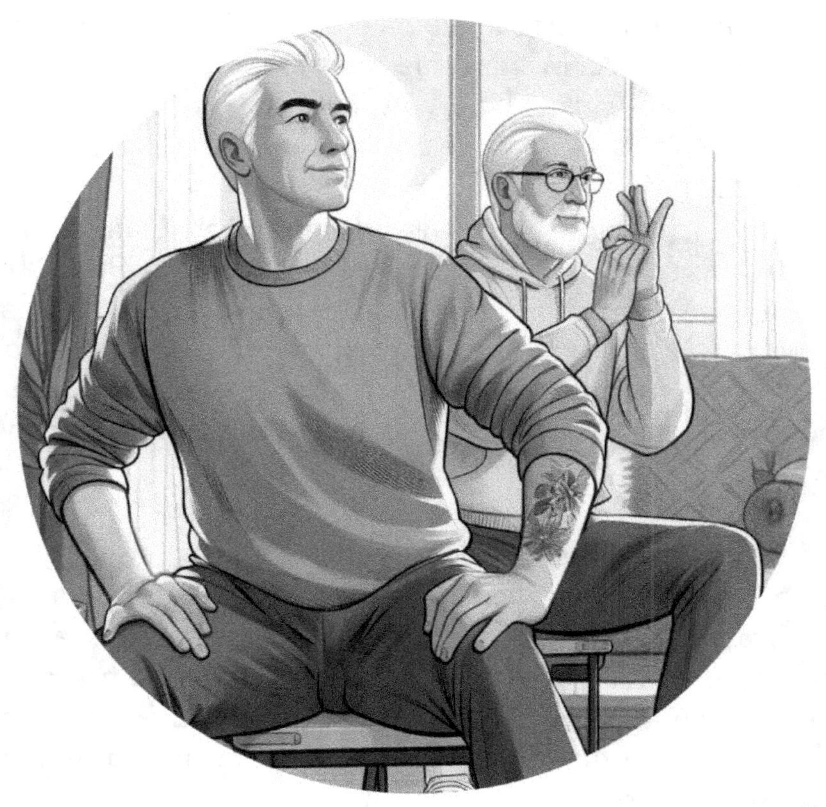

In this chapter, we'll delve deeper into strategies for staying motivated and overcoming challenges in your chair yoga practice. We'll explore various tips for sticking with your practice, dealing with pain and discomfort, creating a supportive yoga community, and celebrating your achievements along the way.

# Tips for Sticking with Your Chair Yoga Practice

Sticking with any new routine, including chair yoga, can be challenging at times. However, with the right strategies and mindset, you can establish a consistent practice that becomes an integral part of your daily life. Here are some tips to help you stay motivated:

### Set Realistic Goals

Setting achievable goals is essential for maintaining motivation in your chair yoga practice. Start by identifying what you hope to accomplish through yoga, whether it's improving flexibility, reducing stress, or increasing strength. Break down your goals into smaller, actionable steps, and celebrate each milestone along the way.

### Create a Routine

Consistency is key to progress in yoga. Set aside dedicated time for your chair yoga practice each day or week, and treat it as you would any other important appointment. Whether it's first thing in the morning, during your lunch break, or before bed, find a time that works best for you and stick to it.

## Stay Consistent

Even on days when you don't feel like practicing, commit to doing at least a few minutes of chair yoga. Consistency is more important than intensity, so focus on showing up on your mat regularly, even if it's just for a short session. Remember that every little bit counts towards building a habit.

## Find Accountability

Partnering with a friend, family member, or online community can provide valuable accountability and support in your yoga journey. Share your goals and progress with someone you trust, and check in regularly to provide encouragement and hold each other accountable. Knowing that someone else is counting on you can help keep you motivated, even on challenging days.

## Mix It Up

Keep your practice interesting by exploring different styles of chair yoga, trying new poses, or incorporating props like yoga blocks or straps for added challenge. Variety not only prevents boredom but also helps target different muscle groups and keeps your body and mind engaged.

## Track Your Progress

Keep a journal or use a tracking app to record your practice sessions, note any improvements or challenges, and track your overall progress over time. Celebrate your achievements, no matter how small, and use setbacks as opportunities for growth and learning.

## Reward Yourself

Celebrate milestones and achievements in your chair yoga practice with small rewards, such as treating yourself to a relaxing bath, enjoying a healthy snack, or indulging in a favorite activity. Rewards can help reinforce positive behavior and keep you motivated to continue progressing in your practice.

# Dealing with Pain and Discomfort

While yoga is generally safe and beneficial for most people, it's essential to listen to your body and practice with awareness to avoid injury. Here are some tips for dealing with pain and discomfort during your chair yoga practice:

## Listen to Your Body

Pay attention to how your body feels during practice and honor its signals. If a pose or movement causes pain or discomfort, ease off or modify as needed. Pushing through pain can lead to injury, so prioritize comfort and safety above all else.

## Modify Poses

Don't be afraid to modify poses to suit your body's needs and limitations. Use props like cushions or blankets for support, or adjust the intensity of stretches to a level that feels comfortable. Chair yoga is highly adaptable, so feel free to make modifications as needed to ensure a safe and enjoyable practice.

## Practice Gentle Self-Care

Incorporate gentle self-care practices like self-massage,

hot/cold therapy, or gentle stretching outside of your chair yoga sessions to alleviate muscle tension and discomfort. Taking care of your body off the mat can help enhance your overall well-being and support your yoga practice.

## Consult a Professional

If you experience persistent or severe pain during practice, consult a healthcare professional or a certified yoga instructor for guidance and personalized modifications. They can help assess your individual needs and provide tailored recommendations to ensure a safe and effective practice.

# Creating a Supportive Yoga Community

Connecting with others who share your interest in yoga can provide valuable support, encouragement, and inspiration on your journey. Here are some ways to create a supportive yoga community:

## Join Online Communities

Connect with like-minded individuals by joining online chair yoga communities or forums where you can share experiences, ask questions, and offer support to others. Online communities provide a sense of belonging and connection, even if you're practicing yoga from the comfort of your own home.

## Attend In-Person Classes

If possible, attend in-person chair yoga classes at a local community center, senior center, or yoga studio to connect with others who share your interest in yoga. In-person classes offer the opportunity to meet fellow practitioners, receive guidance from experienced instructors, and cultivate a sense of community.

## Host Virtual Meetups

Organize virtual meetups with friends, family, or fellow chair yoga enthusiasts for group practice sessions, discussions, or socializing. Virtual meetups provide an opportunity to connect with others in real-time, regardless of geographical location, and foster meaningful relationships within the yoga community.

## Participate in Challenges or Workshops

Take part in chair yoga challenges, workshops, or retreats to deepen your practice, meet new people, and foster a sense of community. Challenges and workshops offer the opportunity to learn from experienced instructors, connect with fellow practitioners, and expand your knowledge and skills in yoga.

## Celebrating Your Achievements

Celebrating your achievements, no matter how small, is essential for maintaining motivation and momentum in your chair yoga practice. Here are some ways to celebrate your successes:

## Acknowledge Progress

Take time to acknowledge and celebrate your achievements, whether it's mastering a challenging pose, increasing flexibility, or committing to a regular practice routine. Recognize the effort and dedication you've put into your chair yoga practice and celebrate each milestone along the way.

## Share Success Stories

Share your success stories and achievements with friends, family, or your yoga community to inspire and motivate others on their own journey. Sharing your experiences can not only celebrate your accomplishments but also inspire others to pursue their goals and dreams.

## Reward Yourself

Treat yourself to a special reward or indulgence as a way of celebrating your hard work and dedication to your chair yoga practice. Whether it's treating yourself to a massage, enjoying a delicious meal, or purchasing a new yoga prop or accessory, find ways to reward yourself for your efforts and achievements.

## Reflect and Set New Goals

Reflect on your achievements and set new goals to continue challenging yourself and expanding your practice. Embrace the journey of growth and self-discovery that comes with consistent dedication to your yoga practice, and use each achievement as a stepping stone towards realizing your full potential.

By incorporating these strategies into your chair yoga practice, you can stay motivated, overcome challenges, and cultivate a supportive community that uplifts and inspires you on your journey towards greater health and well-being. Remember that every step forward, no matter how small, is a cause for celebration and a testament to your commitment to self-care and self-improvement. Keep up the great work!

# Chapter 09

## Chair Yoga Beyond the Basics

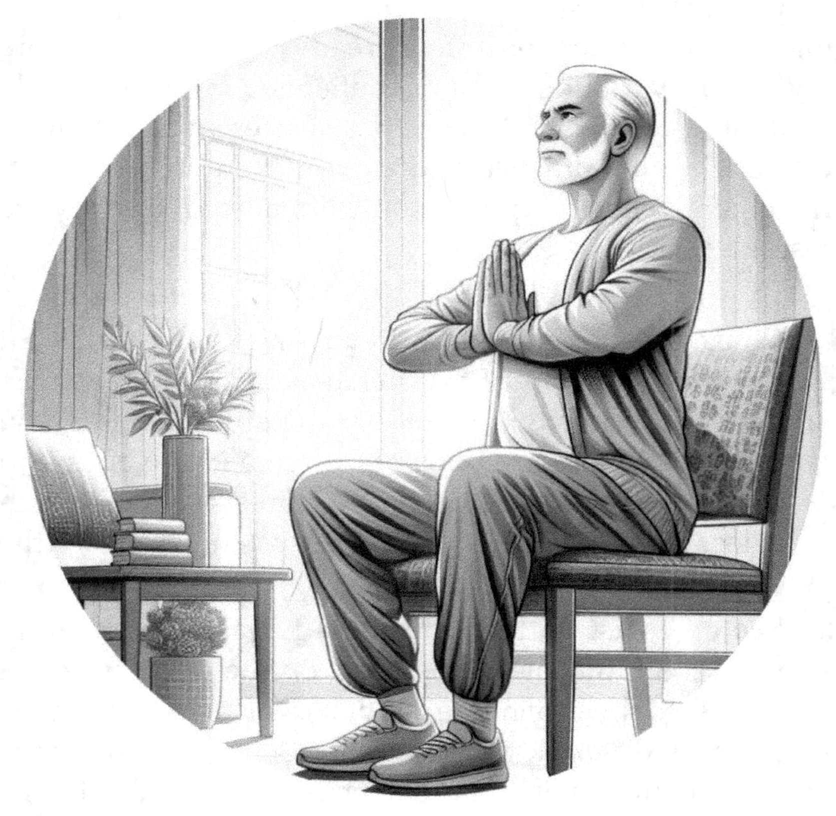

Welcome to Chapter 9 of our guide, where we'll delve deeper into Chair Yoga Beyond the Basics. In this chapter, we'll introduce you to more advanced chair yoga poses, discuss the use of props for added support or challenge, and explore different chair yoga styles such as Yin yoga and Restorative yoga.

# Introduction to More Advanced Chair Yoga Poses

As you become more comfortable with the basic chair yoga poses, you may feel ready to explore more advanced variations that challenge your strength, flexibility, and balance. These poses offer an opportunity to deepen your practice and expand your repertoire of movements. Let's explore some advanced chair yoga poses:

1. **Chair Pigeon Pose (Eka Pada Rajakapotasana):** Sit towards the front of your chair and cross one ankle over the opposite knee. Keep the spine long as you gently lean forward, feeling a stretch in the outer hip of the crossed leg. Hold for 5-10 breaths, then switch sides. This pose helps open the hips and stretches the glutes and piriformis muscles.

2. **Seated Twist with Bind (Bharadvajasana):** Sit tall in your chair and place one hand on the opposite knee. Inhale to lengthen the spine, then exhale to twist towards the back of the chair, reaching the opposite hand behind your back. If possible, bind the hands together. Hold for 5-10 breaths, then repeat on the other side. This pose improves spinal mobility and

stimulates digestion.

3. **Eagle Arms (Garudasana Arms):** Bring your arms out in front of you at shoulder height. Cross one arm over the other, bringing the palms together if possible. Lift the elbows slightly and hold for 5-10 breaths, then switch sides. This pose stretches the shoulders and upper back while improving concentration and focus.

4. **Seated Forward Fold with Twist:** Sit towards the front of your chair with your feet hip-width apart. Inhale to lengthen the spine, then exhale to fold forward, bringing one hand to the opposite ankle and reaching the other arm towards the ceiling. Hold for 5-10 breaths, then switch sides. This pose stretches the hamstrings, spine, and shoulders while stimulating digestion.

5. **Chair Warrior III (Virabhadrasana III):** Sit towards the front of your chair and extend one leg straight back, keeping the toes pointing towards the floor. Engage the core and lift the extended leg to hip height, while simultaneously reaching the arms forward. Hold for 5-10 breaths, then switch sides. This pose strengthens the legs, core, and shoulders while improving balance and focus.

These advanced poses offer a deeper challenge for those looking to expand their chair yoga practice. Remember to listen to your body and only attempt poses that feel safe and comfortable for you. Always approach advanced poses with caution and mindfulness.

# Using Props for Added Support or Challenge

Props can enhance your chair yoga practice by providing support, stability, and additional challenge. Here are some ways to incorporate props into your practice:

## 1. Yoga Blocks

Yoga blocks are versatile props that can be used to modify poses and provide support. Here are some ways to use yoga blocks in chair yoga:

- Place yoga blocks under your feet to provide support and stability in seated poses.
- Use blocks to elevate the floor in forward folds, allowing you to maintain proper alignment and avoid rounding the spine.
- Place blocks between the thighs in seated poses to engage the inner thighs and core muscles.
- Use blocks to support the hands in seated twists, allowing you to maintain length in the spine and deepen the twist without straining.

## 2. Yoga Straps

Yoga straps are useful for extending your reach and deepening stretches in chair yoga. Here are some ways to use yoga straps in your practice:

- Use a yoga strap to reach the foot in seated forward folds, allowing you to maintain length in the spine and avoid rounding the back.

- Use a strap to bind the hands in seated twists, allowing you to deepen the twist and open the chest without straining the shoulders.
- Place a strap around the feet in seated poses to help maintain alignment and stability, especially if you have limited flexibility or mobility.

## 3. Blankets or Cushions

Blankets or cushions can provide additional support and comfort in chair yoga poses. Here are some ways to use blankets or cushions in your practice:

- Fold a blanket or cushion and place it under the hips in seated poses to elevate the pelvis and maintain proper alignment.
- Use blankets or cushions to support the knees in kneeling poses, allowing you to relax into the pose without discomfort.
- Place a blanket or cushion under the head in reclining poses to support the neck and encourage relaxation.

## 4. Resistance Bands

Resistance bands can add strength and challenge to your chair yoga practice. Here are some ways to use resistance bands in your practice:

- Use resistance bands for exercises such as seated rows, bicep curls, and chest presses to strengthen the upper body.
- Wrap a resistance band around the thighs in seated poses to engage the outer thighs and glutes.

- Use resistance bands to add resistance to leg lifts, knee lifts, and other lower body exercises, increasing strength and stability.

By incorporating props into your chair yoga practice, you can customize your experience to suit your individual needs and preferences, ensuring a safe and effective practice on the mat.

# Exploring Different Chair Yoga Styles

While traditional chair yoga focuses primarily on gentle stretches and movements, there are other styles of chair yoga that offer unique benefits and experiences. Let's explore two popular chair yoga styles:

## 1. Yin Yoga

Yin yoga is a slow-paced style of yoga that focuses on holding passive poses for an extended period, typically ranging from 1 to 5 minutes. In chair Yin yoga, poses are adapted to be performed while seated, allowing for deep stretching and relaxation of the muscles and connective tissues. Yin yoga targets the deeper layers of fascia and helps release tension and tightness in the body. It also promotes mindfulness and introspection, making it an excellent practice for stress relief and relaxation.

## 2. Restorative Yoga

Restorative yoga is a deeply relaxing and nurturing style of yoga that utilizes props to support the body in passive poses. In chair restorative yoga, poses are modified to be performed while seated or supported by a chair, allowing for gentle opening and release of tension in the body. Restorative yoga promotes deep relaxation, stress reduction, and rejuvenation of the mind and body. It's an excellent practice for seniors or anyone seeking rest and renewal.

Exploring different chair yoga styles can help you discover new ways to support your physical and mental well-being and deepen your understanding of the practice as a whole. Whether you prefer the slow-paced stretching of Yin yoga or the deep relaxation of Restorative yoga, there's a chair yoga style for everyone.

## Conclusion

In this chapter, we've delved deeper into Chair Yoga Beyond the Basics, introducing more advanced poses, discussing the use of props for added support or challenge, and exploring different chair yoga styles such as Yin yoga and Restorative yoga. Whether you're looking to deepen your practice, challenge yourself physically, or simply explore new avenues of yoga, there are endless possibilities to discover on your chair yoga journey. Remember to approach your practice with an open mind and a sense of curiosity, and to listen to your body's needs as you explore new poses and styles. Enjoy the journey!

# Chapter 10

## The Journey Continues

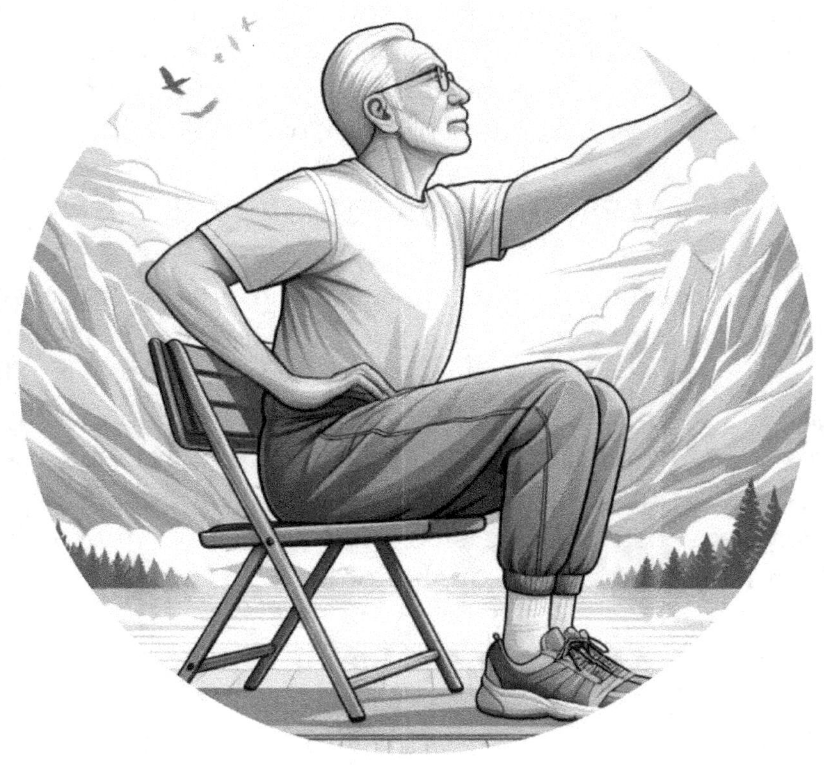

Welcome to Chapter 10 of our guide, where we'll explore the long-term benefits of chair yoga and how to integrate yoga into your daily life. As you continue your journey with chair yoga, it's essential to understand the lasting impact it can have on your physical, mental, and emotional well-being, as well as how to incorporate yoga principles into your everyday routine.

# Long-term Benefits of Chair Yoga

Chair yoga offers a multitude of long-term benefits that extend far beyond the physical aspects of the practice. Here, we'll delve deeper into these benefits and how they can positively impact your life over time.

## 1. Improved Flexibility and Mobility

Regular practice of chair yoga can gradually improve flexibility and mobility throughout the body. As you engage in gentle stretches and movements, you'll gradually lengthen muscles, tendons, and ligaments, increasing your range of motion and reducing stiffness in joints. Improved flexibility and mobility make everyday activities easier and more comfortable, enhancing your overall quality of life.

## 2. Enhanced Strength and Stability

Chair yoga poses are designed to strengthen muscles throughout the body, including the core, arms, legs, and back. Over time, consistent practice leads to increased muscular strength and endurance, which improves posture, balance, and stability. Enhanced strength and stability reduce the risk of falls and injuries, especially in older adults, allowing you to maintain independence and confidence in daily activities.

## 3. Stress Reduction and Relaxation

One of the most significant benefits of chair yoga is its ability to promote relaxation and reduce stress levels. Through deep breathing, mindful movement, and meditation, you'll learn to release tension and calm the mind, leading to a greater sense of peace, clarity, and emotional well-being. Regular practice of chair yoga helps you develop coping mechanisms for managing stress and navigating life's challenges with resilience and grace.

## 4. Pain Management

Chair yoga can be a valuable tool for managing chronic pain conditions such as arthritis, back pain, and fibromyalgia. By gently stretching and strengthening muscles, improving circulation, and promoting relaxation, chair yoga helps alleviate pain and discomfort, enhancing overall quality of life. As you continue to practice, you'll learn to tune into your body's signals and make conscious choices to support your physical well-being.

## 5. Better Sleep

Regular practice of chair yoga can improve sleep quality and duration by reducing stress, calming the nervous system, and promoting relaxation. Incorporating gentle stretches and relaxation techniques before bedtime helps prepare the body and mind for restful sleep, leading to more refreshing and rejuvenating nights. Improved sleep quality enhances mood, cognitive function, and overall vitality, allowing you to wake up feeling refreshed and energized each day.

## 6. Increased Mindfulness and Awareness

Chair yoga encourages present-moment awareness and mindfulness, allowing you to fully engage with your body, breath, and sensations. By cultivating mindfulness on the mat, you'll develop greater self-awareness, emotional resilience, and acceptance, which positively impact all areas of your life. As you continue to practice mindfulness, you'll become more attuned to your thoughts, feelings, and behaviors, leading to greater clarity, insight, and personal growth.

# Integrating Yoga into Your Daily Life

While attending formal chair yoga classes is beneficial, integrating yoga principles into your daily life can amplify the benefits and make yoga a natural part of your routine. Here are practical ways to incorporate yoga into your daily life:

## 1. Mindful Breathing

Practice deep diaphragmatic breathing throughout the day to reduce stress, increase energy, and promote relaxation. Take a few moments to pause and focus on your breath, inhaling deeply through the nose and exhaling fully through the mouth. Deep breathing calms the nervous system, lowers blood pressure, and promotes a sense of calm and well-being.

## 2. Mini Yoga Breaks

Take short breaks throughout the day to stretch and move your body. Perform simple chair yoga poses such as neck rolls, shoulder stretches, and seated twists to release tension, improve circulation, and boost energy levels. Even a few minutes of movement can make a significant difference in how you feel, helping you stay alert, focused, and energized throughout the day.

## 3. Mindful Eating

Practice mindful eating by savoring each bite of your meals and paying attention to the tastes, textures, and sensations in your mouth. Eat slowly, chew your food thoroughly, and notice how different foods affect your body and mood. Cultivating mindfulness around eating helps you develop a healthier relationship with food, make more conscious food choices, and enjoy a greater sense of satisfaction and nourishment.

## 4. Gratitude Practice

Take time each day to cultivate gratitude and appreciation for the blessings in your life. Reflect on the things you're grateful for, whether it's your health, relationships, or simple pleasures like a warm cup of tea or a beautiful sunset. Practicing gratitude shifts your perspective from scarcity to abundance, fosters a sense of contentment and fulfillment, and enhances overall well-being.

## 5. Mindful Movement

Incorporate mindful movement into your daily activities by paying attention to your body and posture as you move throughout the day. Practice good posture, engage your core muscles, and move with intention and awareness, whether you're walking, standing, or sitting. Mindful movement helps prevent injuries, reduce tension, and improve overall body awareness, leading to greater comfort and ease in daily activities.

## 6. Evening Relaxation Routine

Create a calming evening relaxation routine to wind down and prepare for sleep. Incorporate gentle chair yoga stretches, deep breathing exercises, and relaxation techniques such as progressive muscle relaxation or guided meditation to signal to your body and mind that it's time to relax and unwind. Establishing a consistent evening relaxation routine helps you transition from the busyness of the day to a state of relaxation and rest, promoting deeper and more restorative sleep.

By integrating yoga into your daily life in these ways, you can extend the benefits of your chair yoga practice beyond the mat and cultivate a greater sense of well-being and balance in all aspects of your life. As you continue your journey with chair yoga, remember that consistency and mindfulness are key. By practicing regularly, staying present, and cultivating awareness in all that you do, you can experience profound transformation and lasting positive changes in your physical, mental, and emotional health. Embrace the journey, and may your practice of chair yoga bring you peace, joy, and vitality for years to come.

# Conclusion

In this final chapter, we've explored the long-term benefits of chair yoga and how to integrate yoga into your daily life. As you continue your journey with chair yoga, remember that consistency and mindfulness are key. By practicing regularly, staying present, and cultivating awareness in all that you do, you can experience profound transformation and lasting positive changes in your physical, mental, and emotional health. Embrace the journey, and may your practice of chair yoga bring you peace, joy, and vitality for years to come.

# CONCLUSION

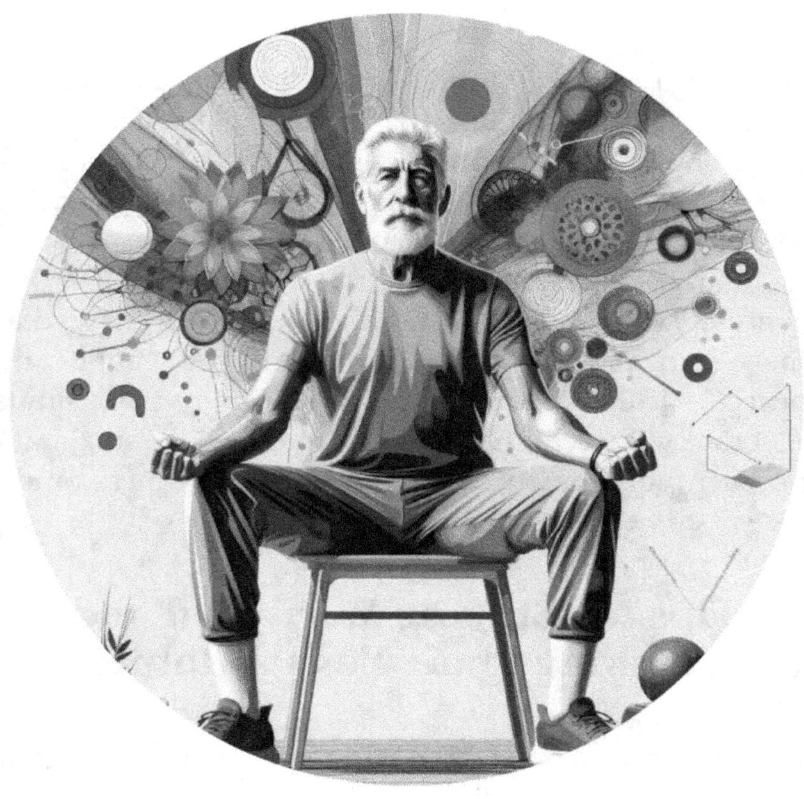

Congratulations on completing "The Ultimate Chair Yoga Guide for Seniors Over 60"! As you wrap up your journey through this guide, take a moment to reflect on how far you've come and the positive changes you've experienced along the way. In this conclusion, we'll offer some final thoughts and words of encouragement, as well as practical tips for staying motivated, progressing your practice, and sharing your chair yoga journey with others.

# Final Thoughts and Words of Encouragement

Chair yoga is a beautiful and accessible practice that offers numerous benefits for seniors over 60. Whether you're looking to improve flexibility, build strength, reduce stress, or simply enhance your overall well-being, chair yoga has something to offer everyone. As you continue your journey with chair yoga, remember that progress is not always linear, and it's okay to have days when your practice feels challenging. Be gentle with yourself, listen to your body, and honor your limits. Celebrate your achievements, no matter how small, and approach your practice with curiosity, openness, and a sense of adventure.

# Tips for Staying Motivated and Making Chair Yoga a Habit

Maintaining a consistent chair yoga practice requires dedication and commitment, but the rewards are well worth the effort. Here are some tips for staying motivated and making chair yoga a habit:

1. **Set Realistic Goals:** Define clear, achievable goals for your chair yoga practice, whether it's improving flexibility, reducing stress, or increasing strength. Break down your goals into smaller, manageable steps, and celebrate your progress along the way.
2. **Create a Routine:** Establish a regular practice

schedule that works for you and stick to it as much as possible. Whether you prefer to practice in the morning, afternoon, or evening, consistency is key to forming a lasting habit.

3. **Find Accountability:** Share your goals and progress with a friend, family member, or fellow yogi who can provide support and encouragement. Accountability partners can help keep you motivated and accountable to your practice.

4. **Stay Flexible:** Be willing to adapt your practice to fit your changing needs and circumstances. If you're short on time, try a shorter practice session or focus on a few key poses. Remember that any amount of practice is better than none.

5. **Explore Variety:** Keep your practice fresh and engaging by exploring different styles of chair yoga, trying new poses, or incorporating props and modifications. Variety not only prevents boredom but also helps target different areas of the body and keep you challenged.

6. **Practice Self-Compassion:** Be kind to yourself on days when your practice feels challenging or you're not able to meet your goals. Remember that progress takes time, and setbacks are a natural part of the journey. Cultivate self-compassion and treat yourself with the same kindness and understanding you would offer to a friend.

## How to Progress Your Chair Yoga Practice

As you become more comfortable with the basic chair yoga poses, you may feel ready to progress your practice and explore more advanced variations. Here are some ways to progress your chair yoga practice:

1. **Challenge Yourself:** Experiment with more challenging poses and sequences that target different areas of the body. Explore standing poses, balance poses, and deeper stretches to continue building strength, flexibility, and balance.
2. **Increase Duration and Intensity:** Gradually increase the duration and intensity of your practice sessions as your strength and stamina improve. Add more repetitions, hold poses for longer periods, or incorporate faster-paced sequences to challenge yourself and elevate your practice to the next level.
3. **Explore New Techniques:** Dive deeper into the principles of breathwork, meditation, and mindfulness to enhance your overall yoga experience. Explore pranayama techniques, meditation practices, and relaxation exercises to cultivate a deeper sense of peace, presence, and well-being.
4. **Seek Guidance:** Consider working with a qualified yoga instructor or attending advanced chair yoga classes to receive personalized guidance and feedback on your practice. A knowledgeable teacher can offer valuable insights, adjustments, and modifications to help you progress safely and effectively.
5. **Listen to Your Body:** Above all, listen to your body and honor its wisdom. Pay attention to how you feel during and after each practice, and adjust your approach accordingly. Respect your body's limitations and boundaries, and avoid pushing yourself beyond what feels comfortable and safe.

# Sharing Your Chair Yoga Journey with Others

Finally, consider sharing your chair yoga journey with others to inspire and uplift those around you. Here are some ways to share your love of chair yoga with others:

1. **Invite Friends and Family:** Encourage friends and family members to join you for a chair yoga class or practice session. Share your experiences and enthusiasm for chair yoga, and invite others to discover the benefits for themselves.
2. **Start a Chair Yoga Group:** Consider starting a chair yoga group in your community or neighborhood. Host weekly or monthly chair yoga sessions in a local park, community center, or senior center to bring people together and promote health and wellness.
3. **Share on Social Media:** Share photos, videos, and stories of your chair yoga practice on social media platforms such as Instagram, Facebook, or YouTube. Use hashtags like #chairyoga, #seniorsyoga, or #yogalife to connect with others who share your passion for yoga and inspire a wider audience.
4. **Volunteer to Teach:** If you feel confident in your chair yoga practice, consider volunteering to teach chair yoga classes at senior centers, retirement communities, or healthcare facilities. Sharing your knowledge and expertise can make a meaningful difference in the lives of others and contribute to the health and well-being of your community.
5. **Lead by Example:** Be a living example of the benefits of chair yoga by embodying the principles of

**mindfulness**, compassion, and self-care in your daily life. By living your yoga off the mat and leading by example, you inspire others to embark on their own journey of health, healing, and self-discovery.

As you continue your chair yoga journey, remember that the most important thing is to enjoy the process and stay connected to the present moment. Chair yoga is not just about physical poses; it's a holistic practice that nourishes the body, mind, and spirit. Embrace the journey with an open heart and a spirit of curiosity, and may your chair yoga practice bring you health, happiness, and fulfillment for years to come.

9 798326 327369